Epilepsy

FOURTH EDITION

Richard Appleton
Consultant Paediatric Neurologist
Alder Hey Children's Hospital, Liverpool

Gus Baker
Senior Lecturer in Neuropsychology

David Chadwick
Professor of Neurology

David Smith
Consultant Neurologist
Department of Neurological Science
University of Liverpool, Liverpool, UK

MARTIN DUNITZ

The views expressed in this publication are those of the authors and not necessarily those of Martin Dunitz Ltd.

© Martin Dunitz Ltd 1991, 1992, 1994, 2001

First published in the United Kingdom
in 1991 by
Martin Dunitz Ltd
7–9 Pratt Street
London NW1 0AE

Tel: +44 (0)207 482 2202
Fax: +44 (0)207 267 0159
E-mail: info.dunitz@tandf.co.uk
Website: http://www.dunitz.co.uk.

First edition 1991
Second edition 1992
Third edition 1994
Fourth edition 2001

A CIP catalogue record for this book is
available from the British Library

ISBN 1–85317–750–4

Distributed in the USA, Canada and Brazil by:
Blackwell Science Inc.
Commerce Place, 350 Main Street
Malden MA 02148, USA
Tel: 1 800 215 1000

Composition by Scribe Design, Gillingham, Kent
Printed and bound in Italy by Printer Trento S.r.l.

Contents

Introduction

Seizures and epilepsy are clinical phenomena resulting from hyperexcitability of the neurones of the cerebral hemispheres. They may be defined in both physiological and clinical terms:

Physiological	Epilepsy is the name for occasional sudden, excessive rapid and local discharges of grey matter (Jackson, 1873).[1]
Clinical	An epileptic seizure is an intermittent, stereotyped disturbance of consciousness, behaviour, emotion, motor function, perception or sensation that on *clinical* grounds results from cortical neuronal discharge. Epilepsy is a condition in which seizures recur, usually spontaneously.

The cellular physiology of epilepsy[2,3]

In both animal models of epilepsy and in humans, cortical neurones exhibit characteristic abnormalities of membrane potential and firing patterns (Figure 1).

The *paroxysmal depolarization shift* (PDS) is an abnormally large prolonged depolarizing post-synaptic potential, which can cause the burst firing of neurones and is capable of subsequently exciting other neurones to adopt a similarly abnormal synchronized pattern of firing. The PDS may result from either imbalance between excitatory (glutamate and aspartate) and inhibitory (GABA-ergic) neurotransmitters or abnormalities of voltage-controlled membrane ion channels.

Figure 1
Schematic presentation of neurophysical events in seizure disorders.
(Reproduced from Ayala et al.*)[4]*

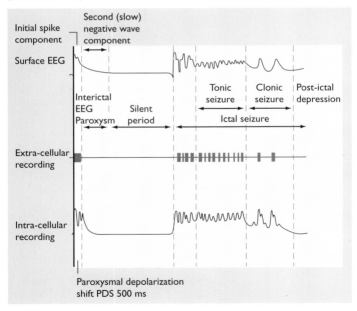

The *epileptic neurone* exhibits abnormal activity characterized by burst firing with intervening prolonged periods of excitability. It may exhibit a pattern spontaneously or in response to afferent stimulation.

Focal epileptogenesis: Within an epileptic focus there is a population of 'pacemaker' neurones that exhibit abnormal burst firing. At these times cells may recruit surrounding neurones into the burst firing. This results in the transition to focal interictal EEG spiking or ictal EEG activity and clinical behaviour, depending on the extent of the pool of neurones recruited.

Generalized epileptogenesis: The traditional concept of a central generator of generalized spike-wave activity (centrencephalic epilepsy) has been discarded. The genesis of spike-and-wave activity occurs in cortical structures, but there is a rapid spread of recurrent excitation (spikes) and inhibition (slow waves) to the whole of both hemispheres via a cortico-reticulo-cortical loop.

Classification of seizures and epilepsy

Seizures are stereotyped within individual patients, but vary between patients. This necessitates a system of classification for both seizures and epileptic syndromes.

Seizures

The most generally accepted classification for seizures is that of the International League Against Epilepsy (1981) (Table 1). Seizures are classified as to whether their onset is focal (partial) or generalized. Partial seizures are further subdivided according to whether consciousness is retained throughout the seizure (simple partial seizure) or impaired at some point (complex partial seizures). Any partial seizure can become secondarily generalized.

Table 1
Classification of seizures.

Partial seizures (seizures beginning locally)

Simple (consciousness not impaired)
    With motor symptoms
    With somatosensory or special sensory symptoms
    With autonomic symptoms
    With psychic symptoms

Complex (with impairment of consciousness)
    Beginning as simple partial seizures, progressing to complex seizures.
    Impairment of consciousness at onset
        1. Impairment of consciousness only
        2. With automatism

Partial seizures becoming secondarily generalized.

Generalized seizures

Absence seizures
    Typical (petit mal)
    Atypical
Myoclonic seizures
Clonic seizures
Tonic seizures
Tonic–clonic seizures
Atonic seizures

(From Commission on Classification and Terminology of the International League Against Epilepsy.)[5]

Epilepsies

This classification of epilepsies (Table 2) recognizes syndromes (Figure 2) that are determined by:

- Seizure types
- Age of onset
- EEG abnormality (ictal and interictal)
- Associated neurological features

These syndromes are important in terms of:

- Predicting prognosis (eg, ease of seizure control and likelihood of spontaneous remission of epilepsy)
- Selecting antiepileptic drug treatment
- Defining the likelihood of identifying an underlying aetiology

Table 2
International League Against Epilepsy classification of epilepsy and epilepsy syndromes.

1. **Localization-related (focal, local, partial) epilepsies and syndromes**
    1.1 Idiopathic (with age-related onset)
        - benign childhood epilepsy with centro-temporal spike
        - childhood epilepsy with occipital paroxysms
        - primary reading epilepsy
    1.2 Symptomatic
        - chronic progressive epilepsia partialis continua of childhood (Kojewnikow's syndrome)
        - syndromes characterized by seizures with specific modes of presentation
    1.3 Cryptogenic (presumed symptomatic but aetiology unknown)

2. **Generalized epilepsies and syndromes**
    2.1 Idiopathic (with age-related onset, listed in order of age)
        - benign neonatal familial convulsions
        - benign neonatal convulsions
        - benign myoclonic epilepsy in infancy
        - childhood absence epilepsy
        - juvenile absence epilepsy
        - juvenile myoclonic epilepsy
        - epilepsy with grand mal (generalized tonic–clonic seizures) on awakening
        - other generalized idiopathic epilepsies not defined above
        - epilepsies with seizures precipitated by specific modes of activation (reflex and reading epilepsies)
    2.2 Cryptogenic or symptomatic (in order of age)
        - West's syndrome
        - Lennox–Gastaut syndrome
        - epilepsy with myoclonic–astatic seizures

           – epilepsy with myoclonic absences
  2.3 Symptomatic
      2.3.1 Non-specific aetiology
             – early myoclonic encephalopathy
             – early infantile epileptic encephalopathy with
                suppression burst
             – other symptomatic generalized epilepsies not
                defined above
      2.3.2 Specific syndromes/aetiologies
             – cerebral malformations
             – inborn errors of metabolism including pyridoxine
                dependency and disorders frequently presenting
                as progressive myoclonic epilepsy

3. Epilepsies and syndromes undetermined, whether focal or generalized
  3.1 With both generalized and focal seizures
        – neonatal seizures
        – severe myoclonic epilepsy in infancy
        – epilepsy with continuous spike-waves during slow wave
          sleep
        – acquired epileptic aphasia (Landau–Kleffner syndrome)
        – other undetermined epilepsies not defined above
  3.2 Without unequivocal generalized or focal features

4. Special syndromes
  4.1 Situation-related seizures
        – febrile convulsions
        – isolated seizures or isolated status epilepticus
        – seizures occurring only when there is an acute
          metabolic or toxic event due to factors such as alcohol,
          drugs, eclampsia, non-ketotic hyperglycemia
        – reflex epilepsy

(From Commission on Classification and Terminology of the International League Against Epilepsy.)[6]

Neonatal seizures

These are discussed in the chapter on 'Specific management problems', p. 70.

Pyridoxine dependency[7]

Rare; onset may occur in utero or after a few months of life, but in over 90 per cent of cases, seizures start in

Figure 2
Main epileptic syndromes of childhood and adolescence.

Neonatal period

Benign familial neonatal convulsions
Early neonatal myoclonic encephalopathy (Ohtahara's syndrome)
Pyridoxine dependency

Infancy

Myoclonic epilepsy – severe
                    – benign
West's syndrome

Early childhood (1–5 years)

Febrile seizures
Lennox–Gastaut syndrome

Later childhood (5–10 years)

Typical absence epilepsy (childhood, <9 years; juvenile, >9 years)
Benign partial epilepsy with rolandic (centro-temporal) spikes
Benign partial epilepsy with occipital spikes/paroxysms
Landau–Kleffner syndrome

Adolescence

Juvenile myoclonic epilepsy (Janz syndrome; may also have an onset
  <10 years of age)
Grand mal seizures on awakening
Typical absence epilepsy of adolescence (juvenile absence)
Benign occipital epilepsy
Mesial temporal epilepsy

the first 24 hours of life. The seizure type is usually generalized (myoclonic, clonic or tonic–clonic), the EEG may be diffusely slow or show a burst–suppression or hypsarrhythmic pattern, and the condition is refractory to all standard antiepileptic drugs (AEDs). Clinical response to intravenous pyridoxine is usually immediate, and normalization of the EEG may also be immediate, although it may be delayed for weeks. Most infants and children show intellectual handicap despite early (including intra-uterine) therapy. Doses of up to 100 mg may be needed to terminate the seizures. A 3-week therapeutic trial of oral pyridoxine should be given whenever the disorder is suspected. Pyridoxine (vitamin B_6) acts as a cofactor for the enzyme glutamic acid decarboxylase in the synthesis of the inhibitory neurotransmitter, GABA. The disorder is probably inherited in an autosomal recessive manner.

Benign familial neonatal convulsions[8]

Rare; usually occur on the second or third day of life, unrelated to any known aetiology. The seizures are mostly generalized, and may be as frequent as 20 per day, usually resolving by 1–6 months of age. Neurological outcome is normal, but one in seven of these infants develop later epilepsy. The disorder results from autosomal dominant inheritance, with a high degree of penetrance. Two genes for this epilepsy have been found to lie on chromosomes 8 and 20[9].

Benign neonatal convulsions ('fifth day fits')

Uncommon, frequently repeated clonic or subtle (eg, apnoeic) seizures occurring around the fifth day of life, in an otherwise normal infant with no known aetiology and no family history of epilepsy. Psychomotor development is normal and there is no association with later epilepsy.

Myoclonic epilepsy in infants

Severe. Rare; otherwise normal infants develop generalized or focal myoclonic seizures in the first year, often in the first few months. They commonly 'present' at 6–12 months with febrile status epilepticus. Psychomotor development is retarded by the second year, and neurological signs may develop. The condition is resistant to treatment and EEG shows generalized spike–wave, photosensitivity and focal abnormalities. Familial cases are common, suggesting an underlying metabolic defect. Structural neuroimaging (CT or MRI) is usually normal but in some children functional neuroimaging with positron emission tomography (PET) may show focal abnormalities. Sodium valproate, clonazepam and the ketogenic diet are the most 'effective' therapies.

Benign.[10] Rare; characterized by brief episodes of generalized myoclonus that occur in the first or second year of life in otherwise normal children, who frequently have a family history of epilepsy. The seizures commonly occur at the onset of, or during, sleep. The seizures are easily controlled and are unaccompanied by other types; generalized tonic–clonic seizures may occur during adolescence. Sodium valproate is the drug of choice.

West's syndrome[11]

The full syndrome comprises an electroclinical trial:

(i)   infantile spasm (flexor, extensor or both) occurring singly or more commonly in clusters of up to 20–50 per cluster);
(ii) hypsarrhythmia on the EEG; and
(iii) developmental delay.

Incidence: 1 in 3000–5000; age at onset: 1–12 months (peak 3–7 months); more common in boys. Spasms may be single and there may be brief momentary head nods, which can be missed by parents and misdiagnosed by doctors. Between 70 and 80 per cent are 'symptomatic' and are due to an identified aetiology. 'Common' causes include: hypoxic–ischaemic (perinatal asphyxial) encephalopathy; cerebral malformations (including tuberous sclerosis); infections (pre- and postnatal meningo-encephalitis); and metabolic disorders (eg, phenylketonuria).

The remaining 20–30 per cent are 'cryptogenic' with no obvious cause and, in this group, 3–5 per cent have a positive family history of infantile spasms. The prognosis is poorer in those with symptomatic spasms and also if the diagnosis (and treatment) is delayed. Infantile spasms are resistant to most anticonvulsants. Vigabatrin or steroids (prednisone; rarely, ACTH) tend to be the treatment of choice—their mechanism of action is unknown. Sodium valproate or nitrazepam are suitable alternatives. Topiramate may be effective in refractory cases.

Lennox–Gastaut syndrome[12]

This syndrome could be regarded as an extension of West's syndrome, occurring between the ages of 1 and 6 years. This is a heterogeneous electroclinical syndrome with the following features:

(i)   'minor' motor seizures — ('stare' (atypical absence), 'jerk' (tonic or less commonly, myoclonic) and 'fall' (atonic, as well as generalized tonic–clonic);
(ii) an EEG that shows slow spike and slow wave (1.5–2.5 Hz); and
(iii) moderate to severe mental handicap in 90 per cent of patients.

Most of the causes of West's syndrome may also produce the Lennox–Gastaut syndrome. Early infantile myoclonic encephalopathy, and West's syndrome, may precede Lennox–Gastaut in up to 50 per cent of children. Seizures are refractory to most AEDs—lamotrigine, sodium valproate, clonazepam and topiramate are the most 'effective' drugs. The ketogenic diet (see p. 90) is of use. Corpus callosotomy may reduce or stop the atonic seizures. Mental handicap is present in between 20 and 60 per cent of patients before the onset of seizures, and uncontrolled seizures or cognitive side-effects of AEDs, or both, produce further severe intellectual deterioration.

Febrile seizures[13]

Convulsions associated with fever occur in 3 per cent of children aged between 12 months and 5 years, without evidence of serious *acute* brain disease (meningitis, encephalitis) or *chronic* brain disorders. Some authors believe that children who are defined as having a febrile seizure must be *normal* neurologically and developmentally, while others consider that minor neurological dysfunction or developmental delay are acceptable. Over 75 per cent are 'simple', brief (lasting less than 15 minutes) and generalized, with no neurological sequelae. The remainder are 'complicated', that is, focal, repetitive or prolonged (even status epilepticus) or with residual neurological signs (eg, Todd's paresis).

The whole concept of what does and does not constitute a febrile seizure and the relationship between 'febrile' seizures and later epilepsy may need to be revised in light of recent information, which has apparently identified a new 'syndrome' of 'generalized epilepsy and febrile seizures plus' (GEFS+).[14] This syndrome may initially present with febrile seizures in the first 2 years of life, before the development of generalized tonic–clonic seizures in later childhood and adult life. The syndrome may be inherited in an autosomal dominant pattern with at least one abnormal gene lying on chromosome 9.

Thirty per cent of children with febrile seizures will have a recurrence, and 1 in 3 of these will have a third seizure. The risk of subsequent epilepsy is 2–5 per cent. Prophylactic AED treatment is controversial, and in most situations, it is not indicated. Rectal diazepam may be used to terminate seizures in children who tend to have recurrent, prolonged seizures. Prophylaxis has *not* been shown to reduce significantly either the rate of recurrence or the development of subsequent non-febrile epilepsy.

Typical absence epilepsy ('petit mal')[15]

This syndrome comprises almost 4 per cent of all childhood epilepsy: age at onset 3–9 (peak 4–8) years; more common in girls. It is characterized by the sudden suppression of mental functioning, with abolition or diminution of responsiveness or memory; the child is motionless with a vacant stare. Recovery is also sudden. Over 90 per cent of seizures last between 5 and 15 seconds. This disturbance of consciousness may be isolated (typical absences) or associated with clonic or automatic motor features (atypical absences). The post-ictal phase is either brief or absent. Whether simple or complex, the absence is accompanied by a characteristic EEG discharge of generalized, symmetrical spike–wave complexes at 3 Hz. The seizures are often unrecognized owing to their brief duration and subtle nature. Control is achieved in 80 per cent of cases, using either sodium valproate or ethosuximide, or both; lamotrigine may also be very effective. Importantly, carbamazepine and vigabatrin may cause a marked deterioration in absences. In up to half of cases, other seizure types (usually generalized tonic–clonic) will subsequently develop; onset of absence seizures after 9 years of age or the occurrence of generalized tonic–clonic seizures at onset predicts a less favourable outcome. Typical absences rarely persist into adult life, and it never commences at this age. Although normal children with typical absence seizures tend to have 'normal intelligence', studies have shown that they frequently experience school difficulties and show a high incidence of psychosocial morbidity; between one-third and one-half of adults who had poorly controlled typical absence epilepsy in childhood experience social maladjustment.

Epilepsy with myoclonic absences

Rare; age of onset; 5–8 years; more common in boys. This condition is characterized by absences with severe bilateral clonic jerks; EEG shows bilateral synchronous and symmetrical discharges of spike-waves at 3 Hz (as in typical absence epilepsy), with retained awareness of the jerks. There is resistance to therapy and prognosis is poor with occasional evolution to other epilepsies, including Lennox–Gastaut syndrome. Valproate, ethosuximide, lamotrigine and clonazepam are the most effective drugs.

Epilepsy with myoclonic–astatic seizures

Rare; age of onset: usually 2–5 years in an otherwise normal child; more common in boys. Occasionally the family history is positive; the seizures are myoclonic, astatic, myoclonic–astatic, absences and tonic–clonic; status epilepticus is common. EEG may show irregular fast spike–wave or polyspike–wave. The course and prognosis are variable, possibly overlapping with the Lennox–Gastaut syndrome. Sodium valproate, lamotrigine and clonazepam are usually effective—but not consistently.

Progressive myoclonic epilepsies[16]

All types are rare. They are frequently resistant to AED medication and are often due to an underlying neuro-degenerative disease.

---

1. Disorders in which clinical presentation is *typically* progressive myoclonic epilepsy:

    Lafora body disease
    Ramsay Hunt syndrome (dyssynergia cerebellaris myoclonica)
    Sialidosis type 1 (cherry red spot myoclonus syndrome)
    Sialidosis type 2
    Mucolipidosis type 1
    Juvenile neuropathic Gaucher's disease (type 3)
    Juvenile neuroaxonal dystrophy

---

2. Disorders in which clinical presentation is *occasionally* progressive myoclonic epilepsy:

Ceroid lipofuscinoses
 – early and late infantile forms
 – early and late juvenile forms
Myoclonic epilepsy with ragged-red fibres ('MERRF')
Huntington's disease
Wilson's disease
Hallervorden–Spatz disease

3. Disorders in which clinical presentation is *atypical* progressive myoclonic epilepsy:

Non-ketotic hyperglycinaemia
Infantile hexosaminidase deficiency
 – Tay–Sachs disease
 – Sandhoff's disease
Biopterin deficiency
Sulphite oxidase deficiency

Landau–Kleffner syndrome[17]

Rare; age of onset: 3–10 years; characterized by near complete or complete loss of previously acquired language *before* the onset of clinical seizures. However, the aphasia may be associated with paroxysmal EEG activity. In 75–80 per cent of cases clinical seizures develop, usually by the age of 10 years, but never after the age of 15 years; these seizures are generalized tonic–clonic or partial motor. Aphasia may be receptive or expressive, or both. Recovery of language is poor and unrelated to clinical or EEG response to anticonvulsants; two-thirds of cases have communication problems in adult life. Psychomotor and behavioural disturbances occur in almost three-quarters of cases (possibly secondary to language difficulties). Pathophysiology of this condition is unknown. Prednisolone, clobazam and vigabatrin may be partly effective. Surgical treatment (sub-pial transection) may be useful in children with persistent and severe language impairment.

Epilepsy with grand mal (generalized tonic–clonic seizures) on awakening[18]

Age of onset: usually in the second decade; over 90 per cent of the seizures occur soon after awakening, whatever the time of the day, and may be precipitated by sleep deprivation. A second seizure peak occurs during relaxation in the evening. Other seizure types are rare (absence or myoclonic). Photosensitivity and a positive family history are common. Prognosis is usually favourable, and intellectual deterioration does not occur. In up to 75 per cent of patients, conventional anticonvulsants (sodium valproate, carbamazepine, or lamotrigine) will control the seizures.

Benign rolandic epilepsy (benign partial epilepsy with centro-temporal spikes)[19]

Age of onset: 2–12 (peak 4–8) years; more common in boys. This is the most common type of partial motor epilepsy in childhood and apparently accounts for 15–20 per cent of all children with epilepsy. Seizure characteristics include unilateral paraesthesiae involving the face (tongue, lips, cheek) and/or unilateral tonic, clonic or tonic–clonic seizures involving the face, lips, tongue, pharyngeal and laryngeal muscles, resulting in speech arrest, dysarthria and drooling. Consciousness is preserved. Seizures usually occur on waking and secondary generalized tonic–clonic convulsions frequently develop, although these are nocturnal. Interictal EEG findings usually show centro-temporal spike or sharp waves and spike and waves are seen during a seizure. Seizures may be very infrequent (50 per cent of patients have fewer than five seizures in total) or they may occur many times a night or day. The response to carbamazepine is excellent and, whether treated or untreated, the seizures and EEG spikes disappear at puberty. Intellectual status and neurological findings are normal.

Childhood epilepsy with occipital paroxysms

Uncommon; age of onset: in the first decade. Seizures may start with visual symptoms (as in migraine) with amaurosis, illusions or hallucinations and are followed by hemiclonic seizures or automatisms. Vomiting is common. In one-quarter of cases, the seizures are followed by a migrainous headache. During eye closure, EEG demonstrates runs of high-amplitude spike and wave or sharp waves recurring rhythmically in the occipital and posterior temporal areas of one or both hemispheres. During a seizure these discharges may spread to the central region. A family history of epilepsy or migraine, or both, is common. Valproate or carbamazepine are effective in controlling the seizures, which may be very infrequent.

Juvenile myoclonic epilepsy (Janz syndrome)[20]

Age of onset: 8–26 (peak 12–16) years; characterized by myoclonic seizures with preserved consciousness that affect mainly the upper limbs. These episodes tend to occur in runs on awakening, or following sleep deprivation, and they may not be recognized, which may lead to the prescription of a wrong antiepileptic drug (specifically carbamazepine, which exacerbates the myoclonic seizures). In 90 per cent of patients, generalized seizures (awakening grand mal) are associated with, and may follow, the myoclonic jerks. In 25 per cent of patients, typical absence seizures (of adolescence) may also occur. Clinical attacks of myoclonus are associated with polyspike and wave discharges on a normal EEG background. Photosensitivity is very common. The response to sodium valproate is excellent, but relapses are common if the drug is withdrawn. Lamotrigine may also be very effective, although it may not be as good as valproate in suppressing myoclonic seizures. Two genes for this syndrome lie on chromosomes 6 and 15, and it is likely that the clinical phenotype of juvenile myoclonic epilepsy is genetically heterogeneous.

Within the past few years there have been reports of new epilepsy 'syndromes'—some distinct with possible genetic markers, others less distinct and currently delineated on the basis of electro-clinical features alone. These include:

(i)   generalized epilepsy and febrile seizures plus (chromosome 9) (see p. 12).

(ii) autosomal-dominant nocturnal frontal lobe epilepsy (chromosome 20q).[21] This has an onset in mid-to-late childhood with clusters of brief, nocturnal motor seizures with hyperkinetic, tonic or dystonic movements but often with retained consciousness; seizures are frequent and may occur between five and 10 times per night. The inter-ictal EEG and neuro-imaging are usually normal, and carbamazepine is generally effective, although seizures may persist throughout life.

(iii) eyelid myoclonia with absences.[22] This is considered to be an absence-related syndrome with an early onset (often under 4 years of age), brief absences with myoclonus of the eyelids or eyes, photosensitivity (which is demonstrable by the age of 4/5 years), persistence into adult life and drug-resistant seizures. A combination of either sodium valproate and lamotrigine or lamotrigine and ethosuximide may provide the most effective control of the seizures.

Aetiology[23]

Unselected population-based studies indicate that the cause of epilepsy is identifiable in approximately 40 per cent of cases. With advances in cerebral imaging and molecular genetics, this figure will increase. The aetiology, however, can often be inferred from clinical information alone.

History taking should include direct questioning about perinatal history and development, prolonged complicated febrile convulsions, previous severe head injury, central nervous system infection, family history of epilepsy and recent development of other neurological symptoms and signs. The age of onset of epilepsy is of particular importance. Epilepsy can be associated with virtually any cerebral pathology (Figure 3), and seizures may occur in response to many systemic disturbances (Table 3).

Figure 3
Causes of seizures and epilepsy by age. (Reproduced from Medical Neurology.)[24]

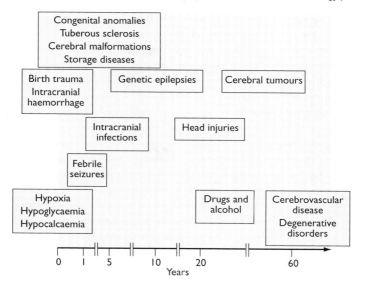

Table 3
Systemic disturbances causing seizures.

Fever Hypoxia Hypoglycaemia Electrolyte imbalance	Drugs Drug withdrawal Toxins
Renal failure Hepatic failure Respiratory failure Hypertension	Pyridoxine deficiency Porphyria Inborn errors of metabolism

Reflex epilepsies[25]

There are a number of epilepsies that are induced or triggered by specific stimuli or situations, some of which may have an obvious psychological component. These include:

- photosensitive epilepsy (flicker- or flash-induced and pattern-induced)
- reading epilepsy
- startle epilepsy
- musicogenic epilepsy
- eating-induced epilepsy
- immersion (hot or cold water)-induced epilepsy
- mathematical- or calculation-induced epilepsy

Photosensitive epilepsy is the most common and the most important in terms of its age of onset and management implications. The peak age of onset is between 12 and 16 years of age and it is more commonly seen in females.

It tends to resolve by the age of 20–25 years, but it may persist throughout life. The precise prevalence of photosensitivity is difficult to determine but one estimate is that it occurs in 2 per cent of patients of all ages who present with seizures and in 10 per cent of patients with seizures who present in the age range of 7–19 years.[26] The idiopathic generalized epilepsies are the epilepsies that characteristically demonstrate photosensitivity, in particular juvenile myoclonic epilepsy, in which photosensitivity may be found in 50 per cent or more of patients, depending upon their age. In photosensitive patients, flickering light of the right intensity and frequency or specific visual patterns produce generalized spike or spike and slow wave discharges on the EEG (the photoparoxysmal response); these discharges may be accompanied by a photoconvulsive response (either a myoclonic or a tonic–clonic seizure).

Sodium valproate appears to be the most effective antiepileptic drug in suppressing photosensitivity, although other drugs may also be of benefit. Data on the role of the new drugs in treating photosensitivity are not yet available.

Epidemiology of epilepsy

Incidence	20–50 per 100,000 per year
Prevalence	4–10 per 1000 (active epilepsy)

The lifetime cumulative incidence of epilepsy, derived from a large population-based study is approximately 3 per cent (Figure 4).[27,28] The discrepancy between lifetime cumulative incidence and prevalence indicates the temporary nature of the condition in many patients.

Mortality: The age-adjusted annual death rate for epilepsy varies widely between countries (0.4–4 per 100,000). This may be due to differences in prevalence rates and/or different methods of recording on death certificates. Factors associated with a higher mortality include:

- Male sex
- Age (<1 or >50 years)
- Marital status (single)
- Certain aetiologies of epilepsy

Figure 4
Incidence, prevalence and cumulative incidence rates for epilepsy in Rochester, Minnesota, USA, 1935–1974. (Reproduced, with permission from Anderson et al.)[27]

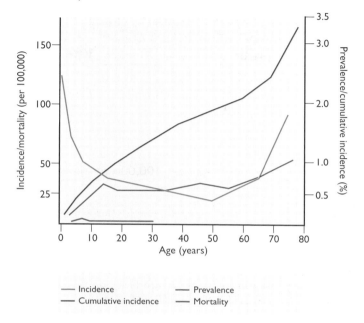

Incidence —— Prevalence
Cumulative incidence —— Mortality

The standardized mortality ratio for epilepsy is high (Table 4).[29] In about 25 per cent of cases death may be related to seizures (status epilepticus, accidental injury and sudden unexplained death). Suicide and cerebral tumours are over-represented as causes of death in people with epilepsy.

Sudden, unexplained death in epilepsy[30] ('SUDEP'), is a phenomenon that is said to be responsible for up to 15 per cent of mortality in epilepsy. The cause or causes remain unknown but may be related to a cardiac dysrhythmia or to respiratory irregularities. The greatest risk (1 in

Table 4
Standardized mortality ratios for patients with epilepsy in the Rochester Study, 1935–1974 by aetiology of epilepsy and follow-up period.

Years of follow-up	Total idiopathic		Neuro-deficit since birth	Potentially acquired secondary epilepsy
0–1	3.8	2.5	20.0	4.3
2–4	2.4	1.7	33.3	2.0
5–9	2.0	2.4	2.0	1.6
10–19	1.4	1.1	6.7	1.1
20–29	2.4	2.0	10.0	3.3
Total	2.3	1.8	11.0	2.2

(From Hauser *et al.*)[29]

200 per annum) is in adult males with tonic–clonic seizures. Low AED levels are often found at post-mortem; it seems to occur less often in children.

Disability in prevalent population: In 1978, the US Commission for Control of Epilepsy and its Consequences[31] attempted to quantify some aspects of disability caused by epilepsy, including the requirements for medical services, the frequency and type of seizures, and the presence of associated handicap. The UK estimates of these variables, derived from a variety of sources, are shown in Table 5.[32] These also give some guide as to the scale of health care required for epilepsy management.

Table 5
The characteristics of epilepsy and medical manpower in a British region of 1,000,000 persons.

Requirement for medical care:	*n*
Cases in institutions, hostels, etc (0.7 per 1000)	700
Cases requiring ongoing medical attention (3.3 per 1000)	3300
Cases requiring occasional medical attention (2.6 per 1000)	2600

Seizure frequency (seizures per year):	Generalized *n*	Partial *n*
One or less per year	450	50
Between one per month and one per year	1650	400
More than one per month	600	950

Associated neurological or psychiatric disorders:	*n*
Epilepsy only	900
Intellectual disability also	1600
Behavioural disability also	1800
Neurological disability also	350

Medical manpower provision (approximate mean figures):	*n*
General practitioners	465
Consultant psychiatrists (mental illness)	22
Consultant general physicians	21
Consultant paediatricians	11
Specialists in community medicine	6
Consultant psychiatrists (mental handicap)	3
Consultant neurologists	3
Consultant neurosurgeons	2
Consultant clinical neurophysiologists	1

(From Shorvon.)[32]

Diagnosis and investigation of epilepsy

Diagnosis

A complete diagnosis of epilepsy requires:

> (i)   differentiation of seizures from other causes of loss of consciousness or altered behaviour (Table 6);
>
> (ii) distinction between unprovoked seizures (epilepsy) and acute symptomatic seizures (see Table 3, p. 20);
>
> (iii) classification of seizures and the epilepsy or epilepsy syndrome; and
>
> (iv) identification of the cause.

Historical information is of paramount importance at each stage of the process and investigations are best deferred until after a confident clinical diagnosis has been made.

The clinical diagnosis is based on a detailed description of events by the patient before, during and after the attacks and, crucially, an adequate eye-witness account. When doubt exists no label should be attached and the clinician should rely on the passage of time and on further descriptions of symptomatic events before making a firm diagnosis. A delay in the diagnosis of genuine epilepsy

Table 6
Differential diagnosis of epilepsy.

Adults	Children

Syncope
Reflex syncope
  Postural
  Psychogenic
  Micturition syncope
  Valsava
Cardiac syncope
  Dysrhythmias (heart
    block,
    tachycardias, etc)
  Valvular disease
    (especially aortic
    stenosis)
  Cardiomyopathies
  Shunts
Perfusion failure
  Hypovolaemia
  Syndrome of
    autonomic failure
 	
Psychogenic attacks
Pseudoseizures
Panic attacks
Hyperventilation
 	
Transient ischaemic attacks
 	
Migraine
 	
Narcolepsy
 	
Hypoglycaemia
	Episodes with altered consciousness
	  Syncope
	  Cyanotic breath-holding attacks
	  Pallid syncopal attacks
	  Night terrors
	  Delirium
	  Migraine (the aura, or confusional
	    and basilar artery variants)
	  Cardiac dysrhythmias (specifically
	    the prolonged QT syndrome and
	    supraventricular tachycardia)
	  Münchausen syndrome by proxy
	
	Episodes without altered consciousness
	  Tics; rhythmic motor habits
	  Shuddering spells
	  Rigors
	  Jitteriness
	  Daydreaming
	  Hypnagogic jerks (sleep
	    myoclonus)
	  Benign paroxysmal
	    choreoathetosis/vertigo
	  Pseudoseizures
	  Gastro-oesophageal reflux
	    (Sandifer's syndrome)
	  Cardiac dysrhythmias
	  Benign myoclonus of infancy
	  Benign sleep myoclonus of
	    infancy
	  Hyperekplexia
	  Münchausen syndrome by proxy

rarely causes harm, but the erroneous diagnosis of epilepsy is associated with psychological and socio-economic consequences, which may be irreversible.

Recognition of seizures

The two most common phenomena causing misdiagnosis in adults are syncope and pseudoseizures. In children, syncope, reflex anoxic seizures and pseudoepileptic seizures are the most common misdiagnoses. Features that differentiate these from epilepsy are detailed in Tables 7 and 8.

The recognition of seizures may be difficult in children, particularly those under the age of 5. Night terrors are relatively common and affect children between the ages 3 and 7–8 years; they occur approximately 1–3 hours after the onset of sleep. Multiple episodes per night do not occur. The child is terrified, often screams, cannot be comforted and usually has no memory of the event; there may also be prominent autonomic symptoms such as sweating and tachycardia. (The main differential

Table 7
The differences between syncope and seizures.

Feature	Syncope	Seizures
Posture	Upright	Any posture
Pallor and sweating	Invariable	Uncommon
Onset	Gradual	Sudden or with aura
Injury	Rare	Not uncommon
Convulsive jerks	Common (myoclonic > clonic)	Common (clonic >> myoclonic)
Incontinence	Rare	Common
Unconsciousness	Seconds	Minutes
Recovery	Rapid	Often slow
Post-ictal confusion	Rare	Common
Frequency	Infrequent	May be frequent
Precipitating factors	Crowded places Lack of food Unpleasant circumstances	Rare

diagnoses of night terrors in children are frontal lobe complex partial seizures; it is common for frontal lobe seizures to occur *many* times per night.)

Table 8
The difference between epileptic seizures and non-epileptic seizures (pseudoseizures).

Features	Epileptic seizure	Pseudoseizure
Onset	Sudden	May be gradual
Retained consciousness in prolonged seizure	Very rare	Common
Pelvic thrusting	Rare	Common
Flailing, thrashing, asynchronous limb movements	Rare	Common
Rolling movements	Rare	Common
Cyanosis	Common	Unusual
Tongue biting and other injury	Common	Less common
Stereotyped attacks	Usual	Uncommon
Duration	Seconds or minutes	Often many minutes
Gaze aversion	Rare	Common
Resistance to passive limb movement or eye opening	Unusual	Common
Prevention of hand flailing on to face	Unusual	Common
Induced by suggestion	Rare	Often
Post-ictal drowsiness or confusion	Usual	Often absent
Ictal EEG abnormality	Almost always	Almost never
Post-ictal EEG abnormal (after seizure with impairment of consciousness)	Usual	Rare

Jitteriness, characteristically a movement phenomenon of the newborn, is frequently confused with a seizure. Tremulousness is the predominant feature, although clonus may also occur. It differs from seizure activity in four ways:

> • It is unaccompanied by ocular phenomena (eye fixation/deviation)
> • It is extremely sensitive to stimuli
> • The dominant movement is tremor (the alternating movements are rhythmic, of equal rate and amplitude; in seizures the movements are clonic with a fast and slow component)
> • The rhythmic movements of the limbs in jitteriness are usually stopped either by holding or by passively flexing the limbs

Münchausen syndrome by proxy is a form of child abuse in which a parent (usually the mother) fabricates symptoms and signs, including 'seizures'.[33]

The aims of investigation of people with suspected epilepsy are to:

(i)   add weight to a clinical diagnosis;
(ii) classify seizures and epileptic syndromes; and
(iii) establish any underlying aetiology.

The use of home, family or even school videos that record 'events' is becoming increasingly useful in the diagnosis of epilepsy in young children.

Investigations

EEG[34,35]

In expert hands the EEG is a useful investigative tool. Among patients in whom a confident clinical diagnosis of epilepsy has been made, a single inter-ictal EEG reveals specific epileptiform discharges always in 35 per cent, sometimes in 50 per cent and never in 15 per cent, while multiple waking and sleeping records increase the sensitivity to 90 per cent. Its main value is in refining the diagnosis (ie, classification), particularly in trance-like states, in which generalized spike and wave indicates absence seizures rather than complex partial seizures, and in tonic–clonic seizures that occur without warning (eg, in sleep), in which the EEG can demonstrate whether seizures are likely to be primary or secondarily generalized.

The role of the EEG in the diagnosis of patients with a working diagnosis of '?funny turns, ?epilepsy' has not been elucidated. However, this role is likely to be limited. A single record is often normal in patients with epilepsy, and non-specific abnormalities and normal phenomena, which are open to misinterpretation, are seen in 15–20 per cent of patients who do not have epilepsy. The fact that a single inter-ictal EEG can neither prove nor disprove the diagnosis of epilepsy is not widely appreciated. EEG is widely available in the UK but only one-quarter of EEG departments are staffed by trained neurophysiologists. Furthermore the majority of EEGs are requested by non-specialists. The combination of inappropriate requests and reporting, out of clinical context, by inadequately trained staff represents a waste of resources and contributes to the misdiagnosis of epilepsy. This is particularly relevant to children and the investigation of paediatric epilepsy.

Imaging[36,37]

The purpose of cerebral imaging is to identify the cause of epilepsy. One-third of patients with epilepsy have idiopathic generalized epilepsy that is caused by genetically determined cortical hyper-excitability in a structurally normal brain. These patients do not require a brain scan.

Two-thirds of patients have partial epilepsy, for which a structural cause should be excluded. CT is abnormal in 15–60 per cent of cases, depending on the selection of populations. In fact, in 10 per cent of cases a single epileptogenic lesion is identified, while in other cases previously unrecognized cerebrovascular disease is discovered and the cause, usually hypertension, can be treated. When epilepsy is unresponsive to AEDs, repeat CT or MRI is indicated, since significant progressive pathology may not be detected by the first CT scan.

MRI is currently reserved for patients whose epilepsy proves refractory to medication; in these patients it has a higher diagnostic yield than CT. It reveals the anatomical extent of lesions and can identify pathology (mesial temporal sclerosis, small tumours, dysplasias) often not detectable on CT.

MRI is rarely performed early in the course of an individual seizure disorder, but a recent publication suggests that it should be the imaging modality of choice in newly diagnosed patients. Although such an approach would probably increase diagnostic yield, management, and outcome, would be likely to be influenced in a small minority of patients only. Furthermore, this approach has implications both for patients (increased waiting times) and for the NHS (costs), which may not be justifiable. Therefore, a selective approach would, arguably, be more appropriate (Figure 5).

Misdiagnosis of epilepsy[38–40]

It is well recognized that 20–25 per cent of adults and children treated with AEDs do not have epilepsy. Incomplete history taking and misinterpretation of non-specific EEG abnormalities and normal phenomena are the main reasons for misdiagnosis. Although drugs are usually stopped with impunity, the resumption of driving

Figure 5
Role of imaging (CT and MRI) in patients with epilepsy: a selective policy.
(BREC, benign rolandic epilepsy of childhood.)

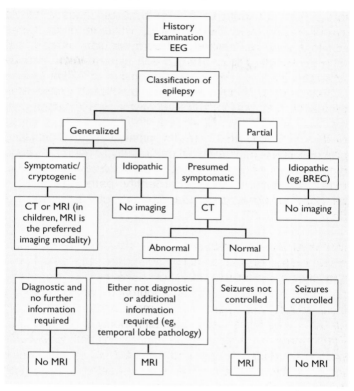

is often delayed and the loss of employment is often irreversible.

At all ages, syncope (faints) (see Table 7) is the most common condition to be mistaken for epilepsy. Doctors commonly fail to ask about the specific circumstances in which faints occur and the clinical features of pre-syncope. Motor (myoclonic jerks, tonic stiffening) and ocular phenomena (eye rolling, eye deviation) commonly occur in syncope but are not well recognized, and doctors frequently misinterpret these features as tonic–clonic seizures. Finally, the loss of consciousness in syncope is usually brief and recovery is rapid.[35]

Patients with pseudoepileptic seizures (pseudoseizures) (see Table 8) are often referred with apparently drug-resistant epilepsy. These events bear a superficial resemblance to tonic–clonic seizures, but are often variable, and eye-witness accounts are usually unconvincing. Review of past medical history often reveals repeated admissions in 'status epilepticus', previous unexplained physical symptoms and psychiatric problems (notably deliberate self-harm). Pseudo seizures rarely occur in boys under 12 years of age and, when they occur in adolescent girls, they tend to develop in someone who already has a diagnosis of epilepsy.

Risks from epilepsy

Children

Perinatal insult.[41–43] The newborn period is the time of life with the highest risk of seizures and epilepsy. The immature and developing brain is susceptible to a number of insults, including:

- Asphyxia (hypoxic–ischaemic encephalopathy)— the most common and also most serious cause of neonatal seizures
- Intra- and periventricular haemorrhage
- Transient metabolic dysfunction (eg, hypoglycaemia, hypocalcaemia, hyponatraemia)
- Sepsis (congenital infection, septicaemia or meningitis)
- Cerebral malformation (dysplasias)
- Trauma (rare, and frequently associated with skull fractures)

The aetiology of the seizures, rather than the seizures themselves, is a more important predictor of permanent brain damage and also of epilepsy. Establishing a useful overall prognosis for a group of newborn infants who have seizures with different seizure types and different aetiologies is impractical and probably impossible. At least one study has attempted to predict epilepsy as an outcome independent of cerebral damage (mental handicap and motor dysfunction). In general, when seizures are the result of an uncomplicated metabolic disturbance such as hypoglycaemia, hypocalcaemia or hyponatraemia, the risk of developing later epilepsy is low and probably no greater than that of the general population. In contrast, when the seizures follow asphyxia or periventricular haemorrhage or are due to a cerebral malformation, then the risk of subsequent epilepsy is much greater. Overall, later epilepsy will develop in 15–20 per cent of infants with neonatal seizures.

Approximately 10 per cent of children with mental handicap and 30 per cent of children with cerebral palsy (particularly the hemiplegic or tetraplegic types) will develop epilepsy, compared to 50–60 per cent of those in whom both conditions co-exist.

Febrile seizures.[44,45] Non-febrile seizures (epilepsy) occur in approximately 2–5 per cent of children with febrile seizures, a rate that is between two and ten times higher than that expected in the general population. A number of risk factors have been identified among children with febrile seizures as being directly related to the later development of epilepsy:

- Presence of developmental abnormalities antedating the first febrile seizure (usually moderately severe developmental abnormalities)
- Epilepsy in a first-degree relative (parent or sibling)
- Complicated febrile seizures (duration longer than 15 minutes, multiple seizures, or focal in nature)

Children with two or more risk factors (6 per cent of the febrile seizure population) have a 10 per cent risk of developing later epilepsy; those with one risk factor have a 2 per cent risk and those with no risk factor (60 per cent of the febrile seizure population) have a 0.9 per cent risk, which is only marginally greater than that for children with no febrile seizure. Most of the afebrile seizures that develop in these children are generalized tonic–clonic seizures, but complex partial seizures of temporal lobe origin may also occur. There is no convincing evidence that prophylaxis (intermittent rectal diazepam or continuous sodium valproate/phenobarbitone or other antiepileptic drugs reduces the risk of developing later epilepsy.

Meningitis and encephalitis.[46–49] Although the most common causes of symptomatic seizures with fever are meningitis and encephalitis, the risks of developing epilepsy as a result of these infections are low. Seizures that occur during the acute illness tend to carry a poorer prognosis, in respect of both neurological handicap and epilepsy. Epilepsy that complicates meningitis or encephalitis, or both, is frequently refractory to treatment.

Meningitis. Later epilepsy is uncommon, occurring in up to 10 per cent of patients. Epilepsy may be up to five times more common in patients who convulse during their acute illness than in those who do not. Beta-haemolytic streptococci and *Streptococcus pneumoniae* tend to be associated with acute seizures (and therefore later epilepsy); this may be related to the age of the child, since it is usually the younger child, including the newborn infant, who is commonly infected with these bacteria.

Encephalitis. The risk of developing later epilepsy (approximately 20 per cent) is greater than in meningitis, presumably as a result of direct cerebral parenchymal damage. Permanent neurological sequelae, including epilepsy, may be seen in 50–90 per cent of survivors of herpes simplex encephalitis and in 30–40 per cent of survivors of measles encephalitis. The congenital meningoencephalitides (eg, Toxoplasmosis, 'Other' (including syphilis), Rubella, Cytomegalovirus and Herpes simplex (TORCH)) are frequently complicated by intractable seizures, including West's syndrome and Lennox–Gastaut syndrome.

Following pertussis immunization.[50,51] The role of pertussis immunization in causing infantile seizures and subsequent epilepsy is unclear and controversial, but it is probably nil. In neurologically normal children the calculated risk of an encephalopathic illness, including seizures after immunization is about 1 in 110,000 injections. The vaccine may simply trigger the onset of seizures in those children in whom epilepsy is destined to develop.

Head injury

Approximately 5 per cent of patients admitted to hospital with non-missile head injury will develop late traumatic epilepsy. Fifty per cent of these will have a first fit in the first year but up to 25 per cent will be delayed beyond 4 years. There are three main factors that significantly increase the risk of late epilepsy (Table 9).[52] When neither a depressed fracture nor an intracranial haematoma has occurred, the risk of late epilepsy is determined mainly by having early seizures (within 1 week of the injury). Where none of these factors is present, a post-traumatic amnesia of more than 24 hours may increase the risk (Table 10).[53] Late epilepsy is more common after missile injury (with an incidence of 50 per cent). There is no evidence that prophylactic administration of AEDs immediately after the injury reduces the risk of developing late epilepsy.

Table 9
Main factors that increase the incidence of late epilepsy in patients with previous head injuries. (Data from patients in a neurosurgical practice.)

Early epilepsy (seizures in first week)	25%
Intracranial haematoma	31%
Depressed fracture	15%

(From Jennett.)[52]

Craniotomy

The risk of seizures after craniotomy varies according to the underlying pathology (Table 11).[54]

Abscess

The risk of seizures in patients with a cerebral abscess requiring surgery is probably greater than 90 per cent, with a continuing risk well beyond 5 years after surgery.

Table 10
Incidence of late seizures. (Data from a community-based series of patients.)

Type of injury	All cases	Incidence (%)
Severe		
Brain contusion, haematoma	154	14
Loss of consciousness for more than 24 hours	41	5
Depressed skull fracture	52	2
Sub-total		11.6
Moderate		
Loss of consciousness lasting between 30 minutes and 24 hours	418	1.8
Basal or linear fracture	442	1.6
Sub-total		1.6
Mild concussion	1640	0.6

(From Annegers *et al.*)[53]

Figure 6
Risks of seizure after stroke. (After Burn.)[55]

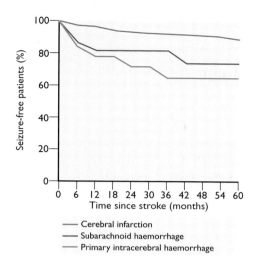

Cerebral infarction
Subarachnoid haemorrhage
Primary intracerebral haemorrhage

Table 11
Non-malignant neurosurgical condition and incidence of seizures.

Non-malignant neurosurgical condition	Incidence of seizures (%)
Vascular	
Anterior cerebral artery aneurysm	21
Middle cerebral artery aneurysm	38
Arteriovenous malformation	50
Spontaneous haematoma	20
Meningioma	22
Abscess	92
Other benign supratentorial tumours	4
Shunting for hydrocephalus	17

(From Foy *et al.*)[54]

Subarachnoid haemorrhage

The risk of seizures after subarachnoid haemorrhage is approximately 20 per cent. If only subarachnoid haemorrhage has occurred, onset of seizures is unlikely after 2 years, but if intracerebral haematoma occurs there is a continuing risk. Risk of epilepsy is greatest after clipping of a middle cerebral artery aneurysm.

Stroke

The risk of epilepsy after stroke varies according to the cause, being greatest after subarachnoid haemorrhage with intracerebral extension of a primary intracerebral haemorrhage (Figure 6).[55] When cerebral infarction occurs, epilepsy is most likely after total anterior circulation infarction.

Drug treatment

Prospective population-based studies have demonstrated that 65–70 per cent of patients attain at least a 5-year remission and that half of these will successfully stop treatment. Thus the long-term prognosis of epilepsy is good for most patients with a short history of seizures. The question arises as to when treatment should be started and when it can be stopped. Is this outlook a reflection of the natural history of the seizures or of the effects of AEDs? Prophylactic treatment has sometimes been advocated before seizures occur. Such prophylactic treatment may be undertaken in patients with a high prospective risk of epilepsy after head injury and craniotomy for various neurosurgical conditions, although no evidence exists that antiepileptic treatment is effective in such cases.

A first seizure. Methodological differences explain the widely varying estimates (between 27 and 71 per cent) of the risk of recurrence after a single seizure (Table 12).[56] Meta-analyses of prospective studies, using first-seizure methods, indicate an overall 2-year risk of 30–40 per cent. The aetiology and the EEG findings are important predictive factors. When these are combined, the lowest risk (24 per cent) is in the cryptogenic group with normal EEG and the highest risk (65 per cent) is in those with a remote neurological insult and an epileptiform EEG.

Table 12
Prognosis for recurrence after 'first' seizure.

Reference	n	Median follow-up	Time at which outcome was ascertained	Recurrence risk (%)
First-seizure methods				
Prospective ascertainment				
Hauser et al	208	> 2 years	5 years	34
Shinner et al	283	2.7 years	4 years	42
Camfield et al	47	1 year	1 year	38
Hopkins et al	306	–	4 years	52
Pearce and Mackintosh	22	> 12 months	1 year	23
Retrospective ascertainment				
Boulloche et al	119	> 5 years	8 years	38
Annegers et al	424	> 2 years	5 years	56
Camfield et al	168	2 years	2 years	52
Elwes et al	133	15 months	3 years	71
Cleland et al	70	4 years	–	39
Hyllested and Pakkenberg	63	> 4 years	–	43
Thomas	48	> 3 years	–	27
Saunders and Marshal	39	2 years	–	33
New-onset epilepsy methods				
Prospective ascertainment				
Blom et al	74	3 years	3 years	58
Retrospective ascertainment				
Hertz et al	435	to age 7 years	at age 7 years	69
Van den Berg and Yerushally	113	to age 5 years	at age 5 years	65

(From Duncan and Shorvon[56]

The influence of therapy on recurrence is not known. A prospective, randomized study of immediate versus delayed treatment in early epilepsy and single seizures (the MRC study of Epilepsy and Single Seizures (MESS)) should clarify this issue and so permit individualized counselling about the need to start treatment.

Untreated epilepsy. Prospective follow-up of patients with untreated epilepsy reveal that the interval between successive tonic-clonic seizures becomes progressively shorter. The risk of recurrence after two tonic-clonic seizures may be as high as 65-70%.

Stopping treatment.[57–59] The fact that AEDs have been associated with various acute and chronic side-effects, teratogenicity and subtle effects on behaviour and cognitive function is an important argument for exploring the possibility of withdrawing drugs in patients who have had a significant period of remission. Against this are the dangers of seizure recurrence, with important consequences for driving and employment.

The overall risk of relapse is about 20 per cent in children and 40 per cent in adults. Most paediatricians suggest a trial withdrawal of AEDs in most children who attain remission (ie, who are free of seizures for at least 2 years). They are concerned with the impact of drugs on cognitive function and behaviour and impressed by the high expectation of success. Adult neurologists tend to be more circumspect, expressing concern over the consequences of seizure recurrence. A prospective, randomized, multicentre study of AED withdrawal in patients who had achieved a 2-year remission showed that the most important factor determining relapse was the cessation of treatment, which was associated with a

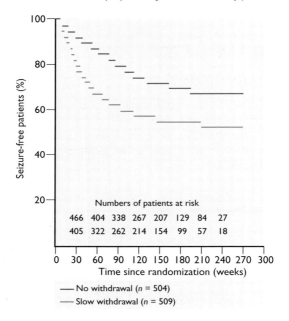

Figure 7
*Probability of remaining seizure-free after withdrawal of drug treatments.
(Reproduced from MRC Antiepileptic Drug Withdrawal Study.)*[58]

two-fold increased risk of relapse (Figure 7). Other
factors influencing relapse include:

- Number of AEDs (one or more than one)
- Whether or not seizures have occurred since start-
  ing therapy
- Duration of remission
- Seizure type (tonic-clonic, myoclonic, other)
- EEG result

Using this information, individualized estimates of risk can be calculated, so permitting informed decision-making about drug withdrawal.

Prognosis of epilepsy

Freedom from seizures

The overall prognosis of epilepsy is good: 20 years after the onset of seizures, 70–80 per cent of patients have been in remission in the previous 5 years and 50 per cent will have been in remission for at least 5 years and no longer taking AEDs.

Reduced seizure severity

In patients with partial epilepsy, in whom total remission is less likely, modification of seizures so that secondary generalized tonic–clonic seizures are prevented and the majority of seizures are only 'auras' without significant impairment of consciousness, may be a more realistic therapeutic goal than total freedom from seizures.

Prognostic factors in epilepsy

A number of factors have an adverse effect on the prognosis for epilepsy:

- Partial rather than primary generalized seizures
- Specific epilepsy syndromes (see p. 5)
- Symptomatic rather than idiopathic epilepsies
- Adult onset rather than childhood (ages 3–12 years) onset
- Increasing frequency and duration of epilepsy before treatment or remission

Intractable epilepsy

Twenty-five per cent of patients have seizures that remain refractory to optimal doses of conventional drugs. The aims of treatment in this group are to:

- Minimize the number of generalized tonic–clonic seizures
- Minimize adverse effects by avoiding polypharmacy
- Limit disability associated with psychosocial consequences of intractable epilepsy—the roles of the clinical psychologist, Disablement Resettlement Officer, social worker, trained counsellors and self-help groups are important.

Monitoring AED treatment[60]

Monitoring blood levels of AEDs in patients with epilepsy has become accepted practice, although it is not always justified. While useful in some circumstances, these investigations can be abused and in some circumstances may be detrimental to patient care. The main indication for blood-level monitoring is the use of phenytoin, whose pharmacokinetic properties are complex (Figure 8). The zero-order kinetics of its metabolism means that there is a narrow margin of safety with the drug, and that there is a good correlation between blood level and symptoms and signs of intoxication. Thus, with this drug, blood levels should be monitored before deciding on any dosage change that might be necessary in the face of continuing seizures. For other drugs, the upper limit of the optimal range is not nearly so well defined. The lower limit of the optimal ranges for AEDs is a meaningless concept. The majority of patients with epilepsy enter remission with blood levels below the stated optimal ranges. On occasion, blood-level monitoring can lead to a patient who is adequately controlled with low blood levels having the

Figure 8
Relationship between dose and serum concentration for phenytoin in two patients.

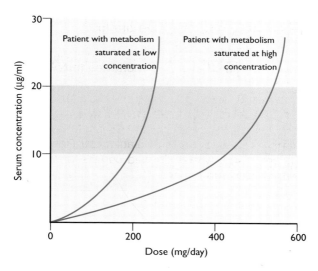

dosage needlessly increased (with extra risk of AED intoxication). Similarly, a patient who needs a high blood level of an AED for adequate seizure control, and who tolerates such high levels, may have dosage needlessly reduced and thereby increasing the risk of seizures.

Choosing drugs[61,62]

Once it has been decided to start treatment, the lowest dose of a single effective drug should be used. The dose of a drug should be increased to the maximum tolerated level before abandoning its use and transferring to another single drug. Polypharmacy is to be avoided whenever possible.

At the start of treatment, patients and relatives must be counselled about the aims of treatment, potential side effects of any antiepileptic drug that is prescribed, the prognosis and duration of expected treatment, and the importance of compliance.

When choosing drugs, several factors need to be considered; the decision determined by individual patient needs.

Major factors	Efficacy Toxicity Womens issues Cost

Minor factors	Ease of use Necessity for serum monitoring

Efficacy[63-67]

There is considerable difficulty in comparing the relative efficacy of AEDs because of the variable severity of epilepsy. At one extreme are patients with mild epilepsy responding to most drugs in low dosage, and at the other extreme are patients with severe epilepsy resistant to all drugs, either singly or in combination.

At present, although evidence from randomized control trials (RCTs) is inconclusive (Figure 9), carbamazepine is accepted as the first-choice drug for partial-onset seizures, and sodium valproate is accepted as the first-choice drug for generalized-onset seizures. An RCT demonstrated that lamotrigine possesses efficacy similar to that of carbamazepine in patients with partial onset seizures, and gabapentin, while slightly less efficacious, appears to be well tolerated. A switch-over to monotherapy study has suggested that topiramate could also be an effective first-line drug. Although scientific comparisons have not been made, there is compelling evidence that

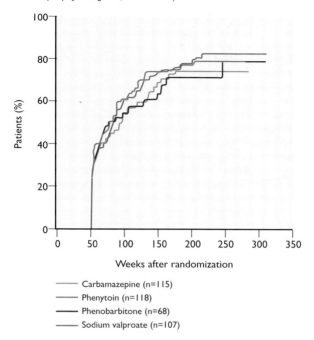

Figure 9
Acturial percentage 1 year remission: all seizures, adults and children with previously treated epilepsy (n=408). (From Heller et al (1989) Abstr. 18th International Epilepsy Congress, New Delhi.)

Weeks after randomization

—— Carbamazepine (n=115)
—— Phenytoin (n=118)
—— Phenobarbitone (n=68)
—— Sodium valproate (n=107)

lamotrigine and topiramate can suppress generalized-onset seizures. Accordingly, the recently commenced SANAD study[67] contains two arms—partial-onset seizures, in which patients are randomized to carbamazepine, lamotrigine, topiramate or gabapentin, and generalized-onset seizures, in which patients are randomized to receive sodium valproate, lamotrigine or topiramate. It is hoped that this study will determine the optimal choice of drugs for patients with epilepsy.

Toxicity

AEDs have several types of toxic effects.

Acute-dose related toxicity. (Table 13.) This is usually a non-specific encephalopathy characterized by nystagmus, ataxia, dysarthria, confusion and drowsiness associated with high blood levels. Phenytoin rarely causes a dose-dependent dyskinesia, whereas an intermittent tremor is a common side-effect of valproate. In children, phenytoin, phenobarbitone and the benzodiazepines may cause impairment of behaviour and cognitive function. Dose-related side effects resolve with reduction of dose.

Acute idiosyncratic toxicity. (See Table 13.) These reactions are rare and unpredictable, and they necessitate immediate withdrawal of the causative drug. Rash, with or without fever, occurs in 2–4 per cent of cases, while Stevens–Johnson syndrome occurs in one patient in 5000–10,000, exposed to carbamazepine, phenytoin, phenobarbitone or lamotrigine. Aplastic anaemia is an extremely rare complication of phenytoin or carbamazepine therapy. Acute liver failure attributable to sodium valproate is almost exclusively seen in children under the age of 3 years with severe neurodevelopmental problems; this effect may be due to an inborn error of metabolism rather than a direct effect of the drug. Felbamate carries a significant risk of fatal haematological or hepatic reactions.

Chronic toxicity. This can affect any system (Table 14). These, particularly the cosmetic effects, tend to be cumulative. High doses and combinations of drugs are best avoided.

A retinopathy that is manifested by a specific, bilateral, concentric visual field defect, which is usually asymptomatic, occurs in one-third or patients exposed to chronic vigabatrin therapy; the incidence may be lower in children. Guidelines on the use of vigabatrin have been disseminated. It should be initiated by a specialist as add-on therapy when all other appropriate treatment options have been exhausted. However, the drug remains as a drug of first choice for treating children who present with infantile spasms. In those patients who are already receiving this drug, individual

Table 13
Acute anticonvulsant toxicity with antiepileptic drug treatment.

Dose-related	
Encephalopathy (tiredness, nystagmus, ataxia, dysarthria, confusional state)	Phenytoin, carbamazepine, phenobarbitone, benzodiazepines, lamotrigine, gabapentin, topiramate
Movement disorder	Phenytoin, gabapentin
Tremor	Valproate
Idiosyncratic	
Hypersensitivity	Phenytoin, carbamazepine, phenobarbitone, lamotrigine
Aplastic anaemia	Felbamate, carbamazepine, phenytoin
Acute hepatitis	Felbamate, valproate, phenytoin, phenobarbitone
?Acute psychosis	Vigabatrin, topiramate

Table 14
Chronic anticonvulsant toxicity with antiepileptic drug treatment.

Nervous system
Memory and cognitive impairment, hyperactivity and behaviour disturbances, pseudodementia, cerebellar atrophy, peripheral neuropathy

Ocular
Retinopathy

Skin
Acne, hirsutism, alopecia, chloasma

Liver
Enzyme induction

Blood
Megaloblastic anaemia, thrombocytopenia, pseudolymphoma

Immune system
IgA deficiency, drug-induced systemic lupus erythematosus

Endocrine system
Decreased thyroxine levels, increased cortisol and sex hormone metabolism

Bone
Osteomalacia

Connective tissue
Gingival hypertrophy, coarsened facial features, Dupuytren's contracture

risk–benefit assessment should be made before and after 6-monthly quantitative perimetry. If there is any evidence of progressive visual field defect the drug should be stopped, because the changes may be irreversible.[68]

Teratogenicity[69,70]

Women with epilepsy account for 0.5 per cent of all pregnancies. While the cause of congenital malformations in these cases is multifactorial (epilepsy, seizures or genetic factors), the risk is directly related to drug burden; monotherapy, dual therapy and polytherapy carrying risks of 4–6 per cent, 7–8 per cent and 15–20 per cent, respectively.

A non-specific fetal anticonvulsant syndrome manifest by facial clefts, distal digital anomalies and mild mental handicap with or without cardiac defects has been attributed to several compounds. The risk of neural tube defects due to carbamazepine is 0.5–1 per cent, while that associated with valproate is considerably higher (at least 2 per cent) and almost certainly dose-related.

Children with fetal valproate syndrome have characteristic dysmorphic features. Neither the % risk of this condition nor whether the presence of these dysmorphic features predict future learning difficulties are known.

Novel drugs are not recommended for pregnant patients. However, thorough pre-clinical evaluation and early clinical data suggest that these drugs may be less teratogenic than conventional drugs.

It must be emphasized that, in most women, uncontrolled epilepsy presents a greater risk than drug treatment both to the pregnancy and to fetal development. Guidelines on the management of pregnant women with epilepsy[71] are given in Table 16 (p. 77).

Carbamazepine

Trade name	Tegretol; Tegretol Retard
Manufacturer	Novartis
Structure	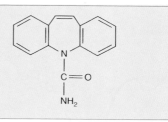
Mode of action	Limits repetitive firing of Na⁺-dependent action potentials
Indications	Drugs of choice: simple and complex partial and tonic–clonic seizures

Dose
  Adults
 	
  Children
	300–600 mg daily; initial dose low with slow increments (NB Autoinduction of metabolism)
	<1 yr 100–200 mg; 1–5 yr 200–400 mg; 5–10 yr 400–600 mg; 10–15 yr 0.6–1 g or commence on 5 mg/kg/day for 10–14 days and then increase to 10 mg/kg/day

Optimal range	4–10 µg/ml (but little evidence to support this)

Side-effects
  Dose-related
 	
  Idiosyncratic
  Chronic toxicity
	Dizziness, double vision, unsteadiness nausea and vomiting
	Rashes, reduced white cell count
	Few known; absence of major effects on intellectual function and behaviour is major benefit

Clobazam	
Trade name	Frisium
Manufacturer	Hoechst
Structure	
Mode of action	Allosteric enhancement of GABA-mediated inhibition
Indications	Occasional use; tonic–clonic and partial seizures particularly perimenstrual. (Value is limited by development of tolerance)
Dose **Adults** **Children**	20–60 mg daily in 2 or 3 doses >3 yr: half adult dose (maximum), although higher doses may be effective and without side-effects
Optimal range	Not routinely measured
Side-effects **Dose-related** **Idiosyncratic** **Chronic toxicity**	Drowsiness and sedation — —

Clonazepam	
Trade name	Rivotril
Manufacturer	Roche
Structure	
Mode of action	Allosteric enhancement of GABA-mediated inhibition
Indications	Drug of choice; status epilepticus. Effective in: absence, myoclonus. Occasional use: tonic–clonic and partial seizures. (Value greatly limited by development of tolerance)
Dose **Adults** **Children**	Orally: 0.5–4 mg 3 times daily in slowly increasing doses \<1 yr 0.5–1 mg/day; 1–5 yr 1–3 mg/day; 6–12 yr 3–6 mg/day or 0.1–0.2 mg/kg/day and usually commence on 0.02 mg/kg/day
Optimal range	Not routinely measured
Side-effects **Dose-related** **Idiosyncratic** **Intravenous administration**	Sedation and drowsiness — Inflammation of veins

Diazepam

Trade name	Valium Diazemuls Stesolid
Manufacturer	Roche KabiVitrum CP Pharmaceuticals
Structure	
Mode of action	Allosteric enhancement of GABA-mediated inhibition
Indications	Drug of choice: status epilepticus; occasional use; absence, myoclonus. (Value limited by development of tolerance)

Dose
  Adults
 	
  Children
	Intravenous; rectal administration may be of value when venous access difficult. Little effect orally
	0.3–0.4 mg/kg (intravenous); 0.5 mg/kg (rectal administration)

Optimal range	Not routinely measured

Side-effects
  Dose-related
  Idiosyncratic
  Chronic toxicity
	
	Sedation
	—
	Habituation

Ethosuximide	
Trade name	Zarontin Emeside
Manufacturer	Parke-Davis Laboratories for Applied Biology
Structure	
Mode of action	? Reduce low threshold calcium current in thalamus ? Enhancement of *non*-GABA-mediated inhibition
Indications	Drug of choice: simple absence; occasional use; myoclonus

Dose
  Adults
  Children
	Up to 2 g/day in 2 or 3 doses
	<6 yr 250 mg/day; >6 yr 0.5–1 g/day or 20–40 mg/kg/day

Optimal range	40–10 µg/ml

Side-effects
  Dose-related
 	
  Idiosyncratic
  Chronic toxicity
	Nausea, drowsiness, dizziness, unsteadiness, may exacerbate tonic–clonic seizures, headache
	Rashes
	—

Felbamate

Trade name	Felbatol in the USA; withdrawn from EU countries in the mid-1990s because of severe adverse effects (fatal aplastic anaemia and hepatitis)
Manufacturer	Wallace
Structure	

$$\text{C}_6\text{H}_5-\overset{\displaystyle \text{CH}_2-\text{OCONH}_2}{\underset{\displaystyle \text{CH}_2-\text{OCONH}_2}{\text{C}-\text{H}}}$$

Mode of action	Uncertain; structurally similar to meprobamate
Indications	Possesses efficacy in partial and generalized-onset seizures, including the Lennox–Gastaut syndrome

Dose
  Adults
  Children
	
	2–3 g/day
	10 mg/kg/day increasing up to a maximum of 30 mg/kg/day

Optimal range	Not yet established

Side-effects
  Dose-related
 	
  Idiosyncratic
 	
  Chronic toxicity
	
	Dose-related nausea, weight loss, insomnia; increases phenytoin but decreases carbamazepine levels
	Skin rash, aplastic anaemia, acute fulminant hepatitis
	Not yet known

Gabapentin

Trade name	Neurontin
Manufacturer	Parke-Davis
Structure	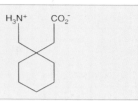
Mode of action	Binds to novel calcium channel receptor sites, possibly related to glutaminergic receptors
Indications	Refractory partial or generalized seizures

Dose
    Adults
    Children
	600–4800 mg/day
	
	>12 yr 300–900 mg/kg/day or 30–50 mg/kg/day

Optimal range	Not yet established

Side-effects
    Dose-related
    Idiosyncratic
    Chronic toxicity
	
	Mild sedation, unsteadiness
	–
	Not yet known

Lamotrigine	
Trade name	Lamictal
Manufacturer	GlaxoWellcome
Structure	
Mode of action	Diminished release of excitatory amino acid (glutamate)
Indications	Monotherapy, or add-on therapy for partial or generalized seizures, including typical/ atypical absences, and the Lennox–Gastaut syndrome

Dose
  Adults
  Children
	100–600 mg/day
	1–3 mg/kg/day (with sodium valproate)
	2–10 mg/kg/day (without sodium valproate)

Optimal range	1–3 µg/ml (half-life is increased by sodium valproate, reduced by enzyme inducers, eg, carbamazepine)

Side-effects
  Dose-related
 	
  Idiosyncratic
  Chronic toxicity
	Mild sedation, blurred vision, ataxia, nausea and vomiting, headache, diplopia
	Rashes
	Not yet known

Oxcarbazepine

Trade name	Trileptal
Manufacturer	Novartis
Structure	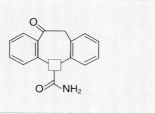
Mode of action	Limits repetitive firing of Na^+-dependent action potential
Indications	Simple, complex partial and secondary generalised tonic–clonic seizures
Dose 　**Adults** 　**Children**	600 mg–2.4 g daily Initial dose 10 mg/kg/day, increasing in 10 mg/kg steps to 40 mg/kg/day
Optimal range	Not routinely measured
Side-effects 　**Dose-related** 　**Idiosyncratic** 　**Chronic toxicity**	Dizziness, diplopia, ataxia, nausea and vomiting; hyponatraemia Rash None known

Phenobarbitone	
Trade name	Gardenal Luminal Prominal
Manufacturer	May & Baker Winthrop Winthrop
Structure	
Mode of action	Enhancement of GABA-mediated inhibition.
Indications	Effective in: tonic, clonic and partial seizures. Occasional use: status epilepticus, absence, myoclonus Rarely used as oral maintenance therapy for chronic epilepsy, particularly in children

Dose
  Adults
 	
  Children
	Up to 200 mg/day in 2 or 3 doses
	
	Usually 3–5 mg/kg/day

Optimal range	15–35 µg/ml; both upper and lower limits modified by development of tolerance

Side-effects
  Dose-related
  Idiosyncratic
  Chronic toxicity
	Drowsinesss, unsteadiness
	Rashes
	Tolerance, habituation, withdrawal seizures. Adverse effects on intellectual function and behaviour

Phenytoin

Trade name	Epanutin
Manufacturer	Parke-Davis
Structure	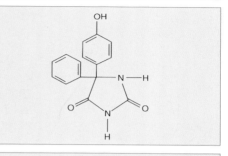
Mode of action	Inhibits sustained repetitive firing effects on Na^+-dependent voltage channels
Indications	Drug occasionally used in tonic–clonic, simple and complex partial seizures
Dose 　Adults 　Children	200–600 mg/day in 1 or 2 doses 3–6 mg/kg/day (higher in neonates)
Optimal range	10–20 µg/ml; the non-linear relationship between dose and serum concentration necessitates frequent blood-level monitoring
Side-effects 　Dose-related 　Idiosyncratic 　Chronic toxicity	Drowsiness, unsteadiness, slurred speech, occasionally abnormal movement disorder Rashes, swelling of lymph glands (pseudolymphoma), hepatitis Gingival hypertrophy, acne, coarsening of facial features, hirsutism, folate deficiency, ?cerebellar atrophy

Primidone	
Trade name	Mysoline
Manufacturer	Astra
Structure	
Mode of action	As phenobarbitone
Indications	Occasional use: tonic–clonic and partial seizures

Dose
  Adults
  Children
	500–1500 mg/day in 2 or 3 doses
	10–30 mg/kg in 2 or 3 doses (rarely used)

Optimal range	As phenobarbitone—to which it is metabolized

Side-effects
  Dose-related
 	
  Idiosyncratic
  Chronic toxicity
	Drowsiness, unsteadiness; often tolerated poorly on initiation and a slow increase in dose advisable
	See phenobarbitone
	See phenobarbitone

Sodium valproate	
Trade name	Epilim; Epilim Chrono
Manufacturer	Sanofi Winthrop
Structure	$CH_3-CH_2-CH_2$ $CH-CO_2^-Na^+$ $CH_3-CH_2-CH_2$
Mode of action	? Enhancement of GABA-mediated inhibition ? Limits sustained repetitive firing of neurones ? Reduced effects of excitatory neurotransmitters
Indications	Drug of choice: idiopathic generalized epilepsies (particularly typical absence, juvenile myoclonic and photosensitive epilepsies), partial and secondary generalized seizures

Dose
  Adults
 	
  Children
	600–3000 mg in 2 or 3 doses
	
	20–60 mg/kg/day (usually 20–30 mg/kg/day)
	A modified release version (Epilim Chrono) may be suitable for once daily administration

Optimal range	Uncertain: blood levels vary considerably during the day and a single specimen is unreliable

Side-effects
  Dose-related
 	
  Idiosyncratic
 	
  Chronic toxicity
	Tremor, irritability, restlessness. Occasionally confusion and/or 'encephalopathy'
	Gastric intolerance, hepatoxicity (mainly infants <3 years old)
	Weight gain; alopecia; dysmenorrhoea and fertility problems

Tiagabine

Trade name	Gabitril
Manufacturer	Sanofi Winthrop
Structure	
Mode of action	Inhibition of GABA re-uptake into presynaptic neurones
Indications	Partial seizures not controlled by other drugs
Dose 　Adults 　Children	30–75 mg/day in 3 doses Optimal range unknown but approximately 0.25–0.75 mg/kg/day
Optimal range	Monitoring not recommended
Side-effects 　Dose-related 　Idiosyncratic 　Chronic toxicity	Central nervous system effects: headache, dizziness, ataxia, tremor, impaired concentration, fatigue, somnolence, nervousness, depressive symptoms and gastrointestinal effects. Recent reports of worsening of complex partial seizures, including complex partial status epilepticus — Not yet known

Topiramate

Trade name	Topamax
Manufacturer	Janssen-Cilag (part of Johnson and Johnson)
Structure	$CH_2OSO_2NH_2$
Mode of action	Na$^+$ channel blockade Enhancement of gabergic activity at GABA-A receptors Inhibition at AMPA–kainate subtype of glutamate receptor
Indications	Possibly drug of first choice for both partial and generalized-onset seizures (adults); add-on therapy in children with partial and generalized seizures and in the Lennox–Gastaut syndrome

Dose
  Adults
  Children
	200–800 mg/day
	3–7 mg/kg/day (given as a twice-daily regime)

Optimal range	Monitoring not recommended

Side-effects
  Dose-related
 	
  Idiosyncratic
  Chronic toxicity
	Impaired concentration, memory and word-finding difficulties, irritability, aggression, anxiety and depression
	Psychotic reactions are rare
	Physical effects include anorexia and weight loss, paraesthesia and gastrointestinal side effects; there is a low incidence (1 per cent) of renal stones

Vigabatrin

Trade name	Sabril
Manufacturer	Hoechst Marion Roussel
Structure	$CH_2{=}CH-CH(NH_2)-CH_2-CH_2-CO_2H$
Mode of action	Enzyme-activated suicidal inhibitor of GABA aminotransaminase
Indications	As monotherapy in the treatment of infantile spasms. Effective in patients with tuberous sclerosis irrespective of seizure type. Last choice in patients with partial seizures not satisfactorily controlled by other drugs. Patients continuing to benefit from vigabatrin require 6-monthly quantitative visual field perimetry
Dose	
Adults	1.5–3 g/day in 1 or 2 doses
Children	3–9 yr 1 g/day / >9 yr 2 g/day or 50–150 mg/kg/day in 2 divided doses in children with infantile spasms
Optimal range	Unrelated to known mode of action
Side-effects	
Dose-related	Transient drowsiness and fatigue, nervousness, irritability, depression, minor cognitive symptoms and headache
Idiosyncratic	Psychotic reactions are seen in <1 per cent of patients exposed to the drug
Chronic toxicity	Asymptomatic and, less commonly, symptomatic retinopathy is seen in one-third of patients on long-term therapy

Drugs in development

Although the overall prognosis of epilepsy is favourable, 20–30 per cent of patients continue to have seizures despite optimal doses of conventional AEDs or suffer unacceptable adverse effects from high-dose polytherapy, and the need for new drugs is well recognized. The conventional drugs were developed on a purely empirical basis, but an increased understanding of the molecular and chemical basis of seizures has resulted in a rational approach to the development of new drugs. An ideal new drug should:

(i) have a known mode of action;
(ii) have either greater efficacy or less toxicity than conventional drugs;
(iii) have simple pharmacokinetics; and
(iv) be available at a cost that does not outweigh these advantages.

Knowledge of the mode of action is useful in terms of predicting the spectrum of efficacy and adverse effects and for planning synergistic, and avoiding disadvantageous drug combinations.

Several new compounds have had a major impact on patient management in the past decade. Lamotrigine and topiramate possess a broad spectrum of efficacy, and gabapentin may be considered as a drug of first choice in partial epilepsy. Unfortunately, felbamate has been withdrawn because of hepatic and bone marrow toxicity. The use of vigabatrin is now severely restricted by the risk of retinopathy, although it remains as a drug of first choice in infantile spasms and in preference to the corticosteroids.

Oxcarbazepine has been available in many European countries for a number of years and has recently received a licence in the UK. Its spectrum of efficacy is similar to carbamazepine and it has pharmacokinetic advantages (no epoxide metabolite, no autoinduction) which suggest it may be better tolerated.

Levetiracetam has yet to receive a licence in the UK; early data suggest that it has a broad spectrum of action against both partial and generalized seizures and an impressive safety profile.

Some of the other new drugs include stiripentol, remacemide, rufinamide, retigabine and zonisamide.

Specific management problems

Neonates[72,73]

The management of seizures in the newborn infant is often difficult.

Diagnosis

Neonatal seizures may be both over- and under-diagnosed. Generalized tonic–clonic seizures do not occur in neonates, most seizures being localized, fragmentary, clonic, tonic, or myoclonic. Many are 'subtle' and consist of abnormal movement patterns (eg, mouthing or chewing, bicycling or boxing, and apnoea) and are frequently unrecognized. However, not all abnormal movements are seizures. This difficulty in seizure recognition is greatest in premature infants. EEG (particularly with simultaneous video-recording of clinical events) may resolve some of this difficulty, but there is an element of 'electroclinical dissociation' in which EEG seizures have an uncertain and inconstant relationship with clinical seizures.

Investigation

The common aetiologies (and time of onset) are multiple (Table 15); in most cases the underlying aetiology can be determined from preceding events, the clinical course, family history and physical examination. If there is no definite history or perinatal asphyxia, an initial 'screen' should be undertaken:

- Blood glucose, calcium, magnesium, electrolytes and acid–base status
- Complete blood count and film
- Cerebrospinal fluid examination (glucose, protein, cell count)
- Cultures of blood, cerebrospinal fluid, urine
- Cranial ultrasonography

Further investigations should be performed, depending upon the clinical indications and results of the initial evaluation:

- Blood ammonia, lactate, urate and liver enzymes
- Blood and urine amino acids; urine organic acids
- Urine-reducing substances; urine sulphite measurement
- TORCH antibody studies (for congenital infection)
- CT of head (for cerebral malformations; MRI is preferred for demonstrating more subtle cerebral dysplasias, but it should be delayed until 10–12 months of age because the pattern of myelination at that age may better identify any dysplasia)
- Diagnostic use of pyridoxine (vitamin B_6)

Treatment

Any underlying aetiology, such as drug withdrawal, electrolyte disturbance or a treatable underlying metabolic disorder, including hypoglycaemia, should be corrected or treated.

Anticonvulsant treatment is virtually always indicated if a correctable metabolic cause is not identified; pyridoxine should be given early if seizures are resistant to

Table 15
Aetiology and onset of neonatal seizures.

Within 24 hours of birth
Perinatal asphyxia
Periventricular haemorrhage
Hypoglycaemia
Sepsis including meningitis
Congenital infection (herpes simplex, rubella, cytomegalovirus,
    toxoplasmosis)
Laceration of tentorium or falx (perinatal trauma)
Cerebral malformation/dysgenesis/dysplasia
Drug withdrawal
Pyridoxine dependency

At 24–72 hours
As for within 24 hours, *plus*:
Metabolic disorders (non-ketotic hyperglycinaemia, urea cycle
    disorders, sulphite oxidase deficiency)
Benign familial (autosomal-dominant) neonatal convulsions
Hypocalcaemia
Cerebral contusion with subdural haemorrhage
Kernicterus

At 1 week
Cerebral malformations/dysgenesis/dysplasia
Herpes simplex (acquired)
Ketotic hyperglycinaemia
Maple syrup urine disease and other metabolic disorders

conventional anticonvulsant therapy. There are incomplete data in a number of aspects of the treatment of neonatal seizures; reasons for this are outlined below.

1. There is no absolute clinical evidence that neonatal seizures produce cerebral damage or are completely harmless. The aetiology of the seizures is more important than the seizures themselves.
2. There is no information on the effects of anticonvulsants on the developing brain.

3. Many pharmacokinetic properties of anticonvulsants (particularly phenytoin) are unique to the neonatal period and this results in problems of either drug efficacy or drug toxicity, or both.
4. The value of anticonvulsant treatment beyond the neonatal period to prevent later epilepsy is unknown.

Phenobarbitone and phenytoin tend to be the first-line anticonvulsants; clonazepam, lorazepam, paraldehyde and lignocaine may also be of benefit.

Children[74–76]

Approximately 50 per cent of epilepsy has an onset or occurs in childhood, usually before 15 years of age, and problems in management are common. Epilepsy is at its most varied in childhood (when there are many epilepsy syndromes and multiple causes), and particular attention needs to be given to making the correct diagnosis (of both epilepsy and the specific epilepsy syndrome) and using the most appropriate treatment.

Important factors in management

1. Ageing and growth have important effects on drug dose requirements and drug metabolism.

2. Duration of anticonvulsant treatment—in most epilepsies this is an arbitrary period, and usually lasts until the patient has been seizure-free for 2 years. Exceptions include neonatal seizures and epilepsy syndromes with known poor prognoses (eg, Lennox–Gastaut syndrome) or high rates of relapse (eg, juvenile myoclonic epilepsy). The EEG tends to be

more useful in predicting recurrence of seizures than in adults, although the decision to withdraw treatment should be based on clinical criteria including the wishes of the child/teenager and his or her parents.

3. Parent and patient education is an essential but frequently neglected aspect of the management of epilepsy in children.

   Important considerations are:

   (i) Explanation of what epilepsy and seizures are, the inheritance and likely prognosis (where possible)

   (ii) Treatment
   - purpose and objectives
   - compliance with drugs
   - side-effects
   - dosage schedules
   - concurrent use with other drugs (eg, paracetamol, antibiotics)

   The emergency treatment of prolonged seizures and intercurrent illnesses must also be discussed.

   (iii) Social implications
   - education (see below)
   - leisure activities
   - employment
   - driving

   (iv) Communication (this cannot be over-emphasized)

| Child Family |
| School doctor Teacher |
| GP Hospital specialist |

Epilepsy may adversely affect family relationships and result in additional psychosocial disturbance. An altered parent–child relationship is a specific problem for parents of children who have their first seizure in early childhood.

Education[77,78]

The interictal function of the developing brain is as important as seizure control and therefore has implications for drug therapy, since all anticonvulsants (particularly phenobarbitone, phenytoin, the benzodiazepines and topiramate) may cause cognitive and behavioural dysfunction. Cognitive dysfunction occurs more commonly when polytherapy is used. Failure in the classroom can lead to failure in occupational performance in later life, while early conduct disturbance may result in adult behavioural problems and a failure to integrate into society.

Learning difficulties[79,80]

The overall incidence of seizures among intellectually impaired and those with learning difficulties is high. The more severe the degree of intellectual impairment, the stronger the association with seizures, and in such cases the condition is more complex and more difficult to treat, and the onset is earlier. Although the aetiology of the epilepsy and any learning difficulties is probably the most

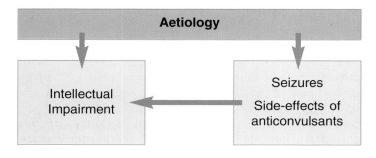

important factor in determining the degree of cognitive dysfunction, it is likely that frequent, uncontrolled seizures contribute to this intellectual impairment.

There are additional problems with the management of seizures in patients with learning difficulties:

1. Seizure control is usually incomplete; in many cases polypharmacy may be necessary, producing increased side-effects.
2. Compliance with anticonvulsant medication.
3. Assessment of seizure control.
4. Assessment of side-effects of drugs (particularly cognitive dysfunction, drowsiness, ataxia).
5. Occurrence and recognition of non-convulsive status epilepticus and non-epileptic seizures (pseudoseizures).

Childbearing years[81]

The oral contraceptive remains the most effective form of contraception. If a patient is taking enzyme-inducing AEDs (eg, barbiturates, phenytoin, carbamazepine, topiramate) then a contraceptive with a higher oestrogen content may be required to prevent contraceptive failure. Sodium valproate, vigabatrin, lamotrigine and gabapentin do not appear to interact with oestrogen metabolism.

It is important to maintain good control of epilepsy throughout pregnancy, and drugs should be continued in patients with recently active epilepsy. Table 16 outlines some suggestions for the care of pregnant women with epilepsy. Pre-conception advice and counselling are particularly important for women with epilepsy who are considering becoming pregnant or who are sexually active.

Table 16
Management of the pregnant epileptic patient

Before pregnancy

1. Consider drug withdrawal where remission >2 years
2. Reduce polypharmacy whenever possible
3. Avoid use of: trimethadione (risk of multiple congenital defects), phenytoin (cleft palate and harelip, cardiac anomalies)
4. If possible use carbamazepine alone (or when necessary for idiopathic generalized epilepsies, valproate)
5. Ensure that folate supplements are given early

During pregnancy

1. Screen pregnancies on valproate for neural tube defects by 16 weeks
2. Monitor blood drug levels during last trimester when they may fall and increased dosage may be necessary
3. Epilepsy may become worse in approximately 25% of patients, improve in 25% and remain unchanged in the remainder

---

After delivery

1. Check blood levels in puerperium and readjust dosage as necessary
2. Administer vitamin K to child at delivery
3. Reassure about breast feeding and drugs

Later life[82]

The specific problems of epilepsy in the elderly include the difficulty in diagnosing a confusional state, which may be caused by seizures; complex partial status may present in this way. As drug metabolism may be impaired in the elderly, there is also an increased likelihood of drug intolerance, particularly to phenytoin.

Management of status epilepticus[83,84]

Status epilepticus can be defined as either a single or recurrent epileptic seizures lasting more than 30 minutes. A practical classification includes the following seizure types:

(i)   tonic–clonic seizures (convulsive status);
(ii) absence seizures;
(iii) myoclonic seizures;
(iv) complex partial seizures; and
(v)   simple partial seizures (epilepsia partialis continua).

Tonic–clonic status epilepticus is a common medical emergency with significant morbidity and mortality. It can be caused by any cerebral pathology, but the causes differ between children (Table 17) and adults (Table 18).

Outcome is determined by aetiology and the time interval between the onset of seizures and commencement of

Table 17
Causes of status epilepticus in children (n = 193).

Idiopathic (*n* = 46)
Seizures occurring in the absence of an acute precipitating neurological insult or systemic metabolic dysfunction

Febrile (*n* = 46)
Seizures provoked by fever alone (temperature >38.4°C). Children of all ages included, as were children with previously abnormal neurological status and children with prior afebrile seizures

Remote symptomatic (*n* = 45)
Seizures occurring without acute provocation in a patient with a prior history of a neurological insult known to be associated with an increased risk of convulsions (eg, stroke, head trauma, meningitis)

Acute symptomatic (*n* = 45)
Seizures occurring in an acute illness (neurological insult or systemic metabolic dysfunction). Also includes abrupt discontinuation of anticonvulsant drugs within 1 week prior to the status epilepticus

Progressive encephalopathy (*n* = 11)
Seizures occurring at any point during a progressive neurological disease (including neurodegenerative diseases, malignancies not in remission and neurocutaneous syndromes)

(From Maytal *et al.*)[85]

Table 18
Causes of status epilepticus in adults (n = 98). (Totals are greater than the number of patients because more than one factor might be present in an individual patient; alcohol abuse occurred with non-compliance in 5 cases).

	Preceding seizure disorder	No previous seizures
Non-compliance	27	–
Alcohol	11	4
Drug overdose	0	10
Stroke	4	11
Metabolic	3	5
Hypoxia	0	4
Tumour	0	4
Trauma	1	2
Infection	0	4
Unknown	11	4

(From Aminoff and Simon.)[83]

effective therapy. Morbidity and mortality are largely caused by an inability of the cerebral circulation to provide adequate substrates for the enhanced demands of continuous neuronal activity. Damage is due to hypoxic–ischaemic insult. Thus paralysis and ventilation without suppression of seizure activity will not prevent neuronal loss.

The aims of management are cessation of seizures, the prevention of complications and the treatment or reversal of the underlying cause. The process of management should be in phases that reflect the underlying pathophysiology.

Figure 10 indicates the principles of management of status epilepticus and the drugs most commonly used. It is now accepted practice to use a short-acting intravenous benzodiazepine bolus and a long-acting phenytoin

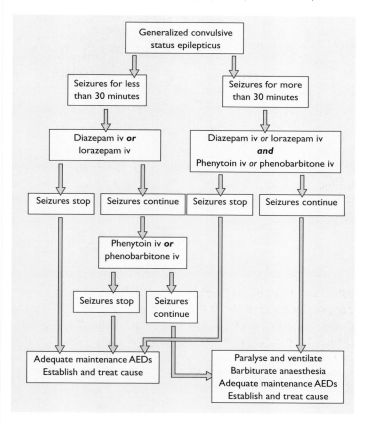

infusion simultaneously when commencing treatment. If status is particularly refractory, the possibility of pseudo-seizures should be considered.[84]

Other drugs may also be indicated, particularly in children when intravenous access may not always be possible

(Table 19). Rectal administration of AEDs is often extremely useful in these situations. When a rapid effect for the termination of prolonged or recurring seizures is desired, lorazepam, paraldehyde, diazepam, or sodium valproate may be used.

Intramuscular administration of paraldehyde should be avoided as it is painful and may be complicated by sterile abscesses, muscle necrosis and irreversible damage to the sciatic nerve.

Drugs can easily be introduced, retained and absorbed from the rectal cavity.[86] Theoretically, the rectal administration of the following drugs can also be used for maintenance therapy; sodium valproate, carbamazepine and phenytoin.

Buccal or intranasal midazolam is an alternative treatment option and may be the preferred choice in some older children for whom rectal diazepam is felt to be inappropriate.

Table 19
Drug choices in the treatment of tonic–clonic status epilepticus. (iv, intravenous; pr, per rectum.)

Stage of status epilepticus	Treatment	
	First choice	Alternatives
Early (0–30 minutes)	Lorazepam (iv) Diazepam (iv or pr)	Midazolam (buccal or intranasal)
Established (30–60 minutes)	Phenytoin (iv) Phenobarbitone (iv)	Fosphenytoin (iv) Chlormethiazole (iv)
Refractory (over 60 minutes)	Thiopentone (iv) Pentobarbitone (iv)	Propofol (iv) (only for adults)

Surgical treatment of epilepsy

Surgical intervention is a realistic therapeutic option for many patients with refractory seizures. A list of commonly performed procedures is shown in Table 20. Resective procedures are intended to be curative, whereas

Table 20
Surgical procedures for refractory seizures.

Functional surgery	Stereotactic lesions
	    Subcortical
	    Temporal
	Disconnection procedures
	    Corpus callosotomy
	    Multiple subpial transections

Resective surgery	Temporal lobe resections
	    Neocorticectomy
	    Anterior temporal lobectomy
	    Amygdalohippocampectomy
	Extratemporal resections
	    Frontal
	    Centro-parietal
	    Occipital
	Major resections
	    Multilobar
	    Hemispherectomy

Table 21
Surgical procedures for refractory seizures.

Rationale	Operation	Indications
Removal of a mass of epileptogenic tissue	Standard anterior temporal lobectomy	Intractable partial epilepsy with seizure onset in the temporal lobe and normal memory function in the contralateral temporal lobe
	Selective amygdalo-hippocampectomy	Intractable partial epilepsy with seizure onset in mesial temporal structures or when contralateral memory function is borderline
Removal of structurally abnormal tissue	Hemispherectomy	Intractable focal +/- generalized seizures in patients with unilateral cerebral pathology and contralateral hemiplegia who have no useful hand function
	Lesionectomy	Refractory seizures caused by focal pathology in resectable cortex
Disconnection procedures (separation of epileptogenic cortex from rest of brain)	Corpus callosotomy	Unilateral cerebral pathology causing a focal epilepsy plus secondary generalized seizures; children with frequent atonic ('drop') seizures with no demonstrable cerebral pathology
	Multiple subpial transections	Intractable partial seizures originating in unresectable foci in primary cortices

functional procedures are essentially palliative. The rationale and indications for these various techniques are described in Table 21.

Focal resections

Any patient who has partial seizures that are refractory to optimal doses of conventional AEDs and whose prognosis for spontaneous recovery is poor should be considered for surgical treatment.

The temporal lobe is the most common source of refractory partial seizures. Although a relatively homogeneous electroclinical temporal lobe syndrome with a specific pathological substrate (mesial temporal sclerosis) has been identified, this is not the case for extratemporal seizures. Unlike seizures of frontal lobe origin, temporal lobe seizures are easy to lateralize and, unlike the parietal and occipital lobes, the temporal lobe can be removed with relative impunity. Consequently temporal lobe resections account for approximately two-thirds of all operations performed for intractable epilepsy.

There are no accurate estimates of how many patients might benefit from temporal lobe surgery. However, the available epidemiological data suggests that, in the UK, there is a reservoir of approximately 16,000 patients who have a history consistent with mesial temporal sclerosis and that about 1000 new patients per year may present with this condition and epilepsy that subsequently proves to be resistant to drug treatment. In addition there are several thousand patients with definable structural abnormalities, mainly indolent tumours. Despite these figures, only 400 temporal lobe resections were performed in the UK in 1998. This situation is likely to improve as more neuroscience centres develop and establish epilepsy surgery programmes.

Pre-surgical evaluation

A patient must fulfil certain criteria if surgery is to be considered.

1. The patient must benefit from cure of the epilepsy—this is less likely if:

   (i)   the epilepsy is not the main cause of disability;
   (ii) the IQ is less than 70; and
   (iii) the age is over 50 (the second decade is the optimal time for consideration of surgical treatment).

2. The site of seizure onset can be defined using imaging techniques, or, in the absence of structural pathology, by electrophysiological methods. Although conventional CT can detect gross pathology, it has been superseded by MRI, which is superior at detecting small structural and atrophic lesions (Figures 11 and 12). Asymmetry of mesial temporal structures, demonstrated by high-definition MRI (volumes, T_2 relaxation times, FLAIR sequences) is highly correlated with histopathology and post-operative outcome. The role of functional imaging techniques is becoming clearer.

Positron emission tomography (PET) scanning demonstrates hypometabolism in epileptic foci inter-ictally and is a reliable indicator of the site of epileptogenic lesions. However, PET scanners are expensive to install and operate, and ictal events cannot easily be recorded with this technique. Consequently this instrument is not likely to become generally available. HMPAO single photon emission computerized tomography (SPECT) scans reveal hypoperfusion in epileptic foci inter-ictally and hyperperfusion post-ictally.

A comparison between inter-ictal and ictal SPECT (Figure 13) is highly predictive of the seizure focus. In some centres concordance between inter-ictal EEG, MRI, SPECT and psychometry obviates the need for invasive ictal monitoring.

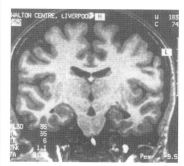

Figure 11
MR scan showing atrophy of the left temporal lobe.

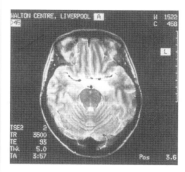

Figure 12
Left mesial temporal high-density lesion.

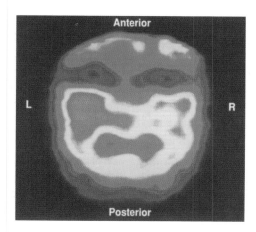

Figure 13
Ictal HMPAO-SPECT scan showing left temporal hyperperfusion extending into the basal ganglia and adjacent frontal lobe. This is a typical pattern seen in seizures of mesial temporal origin. (Reproduced with the kind permission of Dr R Duncan and Dr P Chauvel, Rennes, France.)

The EEG remains the primary means of pre-operative localization. A well-localized inter-ictal anterior temporal spike focus provides useful localizing information. However, bilateral, independent spike foci are common and unilateral foci may be falsely lateralizing. Multi-contact foramen ovale electrodes are now accepted as a useful method for lateralizing seizures that have a suspected medial temporal onset. Subdural and depth or intra-cerebral electrodes provide means of recording from large areas of cortex and are probably best reserved for differentiating between temporal and extra-temporal seizure onsets.

3. Overall cerebral functioning and, in particular, the functional importance of the side of proposed resection must be assessed.

Baseline neuropsychological evaluation involves a series of paper and pencil tests of intellect and memory. Verbal IQ and memory are left hemisphere functions, whereas performance IQ and visual memory are right hemisphere functions. A significant difference between verbal and visual scores may provide evidence of dysfunction in either temporal lobe. An IQ of less than 70 indicates generalized intellectual impairment and may be a contra-indication to focal resection.

The intra-carotid amytal (WADA) test was originally designed to lateralize speech function. It is used to determine if the temporal lobe contralateral to that of proposed surgical resection can sustain memory independently. Furthermore, memory impairment ipsilateral to the side of seizure onset suggests functional impairment in an epileptogenic temporal lobe. Pre-surgical investigation protocols have varied considerably between centres but there is increasing agreement on a relatively non-invasive approach. Concordance between tests increases the chance of surgical success. The protocol used in Liverpool is shown in Figure 14.

Figure 14
Example of a pre-surgical investigation protocol. (WADA test, intra-carotid amytal test named after Dr Juhn Wada, who designed the procedure.)

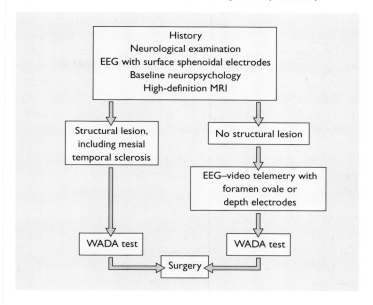

Surgical outcome

Recent advances in pre-surgical investigation protocols and operative techniques have resulted in a rapid expansion of neuroscience centres performing epilepsy surgery in Europe and USA. Consequently the absolute number, and the proportion, of successfully treated cases is steadily rising (Tables 22, 23 and 24).

Overall mortality is less than 1 per cent and operative morbidity (hemiplegia, hemianopia) is 3–4 per cent.

Table 22
Outcome for limbic resections. (ATL, anterior temporal lobectomy; AH, amygdalohippocampectomy.) (Reproduced from Engel,[87] with permission.)

	Before 1985 %		1986–1990 ATL (%)		AH (%)	
Seizure-free	1296	(55.5)	2429	(67.9)	284	(68.8)
Improved	648	(27.7)	860	(24.0)	92	(22.3)
Not improved	392	(16.8)	290	(8.1)	37	(9.0)
Total	2336	(100)	3579	(100)	413	(100)

Table 23
Outcome for neocortical resections. (ETR, extratemporal resection; L, lesionectomy.) (Reproduced from Engel,[87] with permission.)

	Before 1985 %		1986–1990 ETR (%)		L (%)	
Seizure-free	356	(43.2)	363	(45.1)	195	(66.6)
Improved	229	(27.8)	283	(35.2)	63	(21.5)
Not improved	240	(29.1)	159	(19.8)	35	(11.9)
Total	825	(100)	805	(100)	293	(100)

Table 24
Outcome for hemispheric removals. (H, hemispherectomy; MR, large multilobar resection.) (Reproduced from Engel,[87] with permission.)

	Before 1985 %		1986–1990 H (%)		MR (%)	
Seizure-free	68	(77.3)	128	(67.4)	75	(45.2)
Improved	16	(18.2)	40	(21.1)	59	(35.5)
Not improved	4	(4.5)	22	(11.6)	32	(19.3)
Total	88	(100)	190	(100)	166	(100)

Other treatments

Many different approaches to the treatment of epilepsy have been tried, including dietary manipulation, vagal nerve stimulation and behaviour modification:

Dietary modification	Ketogenic diet Oligoantigenic diet (allergy-avoiding diet)
Physical treatment	Stimulation of the vagus nerve
Drugs	Immunoglobulins (intravenous) Vitamin C Vitamin D Vitamin E
Behavioural modifications	Avoidance of seizure-inducing factors

Dietary modification[88,89]

Ketogenic diet.[89,90] This has been used for many years in the treatment of refractory seizures of all types and aetiologies. Major problems with the diet include its unpalatability and the need for obsessional adherence; motivation and compliance may therefore be limited. Diarrhoea, vitamin and iron deficiencies and altered platelet function are additional problems. Practical methods of maintaining a successful ketogenic diet include the use of medium-chain triglycerides to improve the palatability of the diet, and the advice of an enthusiastic and preferably experienced dietitian. Fat or medium-chain triglycerides provides 80 per cent of calories; carbohydrate intake is low, and vitamin and mineral supplements must be given. The degree of success achieved varies considerably and may be a reflection both of doctors' attitudes and of patients' compliance. The diet should be followed strictly for at least 4–6 weeks before a decision is made as to whether it has been effective. To be of maximum benefit, the diet should last for relatively short periods of between 3 and 12 months. No controlled data on the value of such a diet are currently available, and the precise mechanism of action is unknown, although it seems to be related to a high concentration of ketone bodies in the blood.

Physical treatment

Vagal nerve stimulation.[91,92] The mechanism of action whereby stimulation of the vagus nerve leads to inhibition of seizures is uncertain. The procedure involves implanting a programmable generator (resembling a cardiac pacemaker) beneath the left clavicle with the stimulating electrodes wrapped around the left vagus nerve. It remains to be determined which specific seizure types show the best response and which patients (of all ages) derive the most benefit. Hoarseness, dyspnea and localized infection are the most common side-effects. A national, randomized controlled trial against one or more antiepileptic drugs is currently being planned.

Drugs[93,94]

Immunoglobulins. Anecdotal reports suggest that 2- or 3-weekly infusions of intravenous immunoglobulins may be of value in the treatment of intractable seizures in certain patients (particularly those with myoclonic seizures or certain immune deficiencies (eg, IgG2 deficiency). The underlying basis for their action is unknown and as yet there has been no satisfactory placebo-controlled study. The early use of immunoglobulins may be worth considering in those children who present with an acute epileptic encephalopathy, including the Lennox–Gastaut syndrome.

Behaviour therapy[95,96]

This includes the important approach of avoiding or regulating seizure-precipitating (inducing) factors, the most common of which are photic stimuli.

The psychiatric and psychological aspects of epilepsy

The most serious aspect of epilepsy is sometimes not the seizure itself but the associated psychiatric and psychosocial consequences. An increasing number of studies have documented evidence of an increased incidence of psychiatric and psychological disturbances in populations of people with epilepsy, including psychosis, aggression, sexual dysfunction, affective disorders, personality and behaviour changes and general psychopathology.[97] In addition, patients with epilepsy also have to contend with a secondary psychosocial effect, which may include unemployment, perceived stigma and actual discrimination, limited social contacts, low levels of self-esteem and lack of financial resources.

A classification of the psychiatric and psychological consequences is shown in Table 25.

Psychiatric disorder and underlying causes in epilepsy

Cognitive, behavioural, emotional and psychiatric disturbances can be observed in patients who present with seizures when the underlying cause for the disturbances may be due to an organic brain syndrome or brain pathology of unknown

Table 25
Associations between epilepsy and psychological disturbances.

1. **Psychiatric disorder associated with the underlying cause**
2. **Behavioural disturbances associated with the seizure**
   - Pre-ictal
   - Ictal
   - Post-ictal
3. **Interictal**
   - Cognitive
   - Personality
   - Sexual behaviour
   - Emotional disorder
   - Psychosis

origin rather than to the epilepsy. It is not uncommon for adults and children with a mental handicap to present with both atypical psychosis and seizures.

Behavioural disturbances associated with the seizure

Several phenomena have been associated with the pre-ictal and post-ictal stages of seizure. A pre-ictal or pro-dromal phenomenon that presents as increased anxiety, tension, irritability and dysphoria may occur several days before a seizure but then disappear after the attack. Psychiatric disturbances (including changes in memory, ideation and affect, illusions and hallucinations and autonomic behaviour) can also occur during and after the seizure. These disturbances have been primarily associated with complex partial seizures.

Interictal psychosis

There is evidence arising from several different studies that patients with epilepsy are more at risk of developing psychoses. Recent research has associated psychosis with temporal lobe epilepsy (TLE), while other research has implicated the activity of certain brain structures, including the basal ganglia and the limbic system.

Epilepsy and sexual behaviour

A number of studies have investigated the relationship between sexual behaviour and epilepsy. One reason for this is the concern that sexual intercourse may bring on a seizure. The major conclusions from these studies suggest that patients with TLE have significantly higher incidence of hyposexuality than patients with generalized epilepsies. Psychological and social factors must also be expected to contribute to the relationship between sexual behaviour and epilepsy, especially in terms of the overall effects of low self-esteem, anxiety and depression and unemployment.

Epilepsy and emotional disorder

Mood disorders, predominantly anxiety and depression, occur frequently in people with epilepsy. A number of factors have been linked to the pathogenesis of depression including patients' fears, social stigmatization, adverse life events and a past history of depression. Disturbances in the physical, psychological and social aspects of patients with epilepsy often result in depression. The incidence of suicide has been estimated to be four or five times greater than it is in the general population, and more than 25 times higher in patients with TLE.

Epilepsy and personality

Recent research has discredited the notion of an epileptic personality, and personality difficulties per se have been found to exist in only a minority of patients with epilepsy. Lesions in the temporal lobe have been associated with abnormalities of personality, including increased levels of depression, aggression and mood instability. However, psychological and social factors, including low self-esteem, social isolation and real and perceived stigmatization, have also been implicated in the development of personality disturbances.

Epilepsy and cognition

Early research associated epilepsy with intellectual decline. However, it is well established that only a very small minority of patients with epilepsy show changes in cognitive functioning. Cognitive changes, including intellect, memory and language, have been associated with brain damage, adverse effects of AEDs in high doses and periods of recurrent and frequent abnormal electrical activity.

Epilepsy and social restrictions

Active epilepsy impairs all aspects of a social adjustment in children and adults. There is well-documented evidence that seizure onset in childhood has implications for learning, behaviour, personality development and acquisition of the social skills required for normal functioning in adult life.

Adults with epilepsy are often less well equipped than their non-epileptic peers to develop relationships and to compete in the job market.

These problems are exacerbated by the attitudes of the patients themselves (adjustment to seizures and perception of stigma), of parents (over-protectiveness), of peers (ignorance and rejection) and of society (restrictions, both legal and discriminatory).

These social difficulties are clearly inter-related and are probably important in the aetiology of psychological consequences, although this issue has not been satisfactorily investigated.[98]

Patient's perceived impact of epilepsy

There have been a number of studies that suggest that people with epilepsy suffer significant psychosocial problems in comparison with people without epilepsy. Most of these studies, however, have been hospital based and as a consequence have involved patients with more difficult-to-manage epilepsy, resulting in a much more negative profile.

A study of people with epilepsy in remission reported a much more positive profile among that group than in patients with frequent seizures. A recent community study examining the relationship between the frequency of seizures with psychosocial functioning (using a patient-based measure of the perceived impact of epilepsy) revealed a clear linear relationship. A similar result was reported from the same study when it was found that the severity of seizures was related to psychosocial functioning—the more frequent and more severe the seizures, the more likely patients were to report problems with aspects of their psychosocial functioning (Table 26).

Conclusions

The diagnosis of epilepsy has wider implications than just the medical management of seizures. There is well-documented evidence of the social and psychological consequences of epilepsy. It is therefore important in the management of patients with epilepsy to consider not only the seizures themselves but also the consequences of those seizures on the patients' overall quality of life.

Table 26

Perceived impact of epilepsy and treatment by seizure frequency. (Figures are the percentage of patients who believed that their epilepsy or their treatment had had either some effect or a lot of effect on the factor listed.)

Factor	Seizure frequency		
	None in past year (%)	Less than one per month (%)	At least one per month (%)
Relationship with other close family members	16	23	37
Social life and activities	26	39	57
Ability to work in paid employment	24	34	54
Health overall	22	31	47
Relationships with friends	15	25	40
Feelings about self	29	39	51
Plans and ambitions for the future	33	44	63
Standard of living	23	34	50

Restrictions for people with epilepsy

Employment

In certain areas of employment, there are a number of barriers facing epileptic patients. Some of these barriers are statutory (Table 27), but some are discriminatory and potentially amenable to change.[99]

Driving

Adults with epilepsy need careful counselling about driving. Those with a history of epilepsy may only drive if:

(i) they have had no epileptic seizures of any kind for 1 year;[100]

or

(ii) any seizures they have had preceding application have been during sleep, the first sleep seizure succeeding the last awakening seizure by at least 3 years before the application;

and

(iii) driving is not likely to be a source of danger to the public.

Table 27
Some occupations affected by statutory barriers.

Occupation	Regulations
Aircraft pilot	Applicants shall have no established medical history of clinical diagnosis of epilepsy
Ambulance driver	Barrier if seizure occurred since age of 5 for drivers or crew. Clerical work available to those who develop epilepsy in employment
Armed services Army	Applicants are rejected on grounds of epilepsy and are likely to be discharged if they develop epilepsy during employment. For those who have had no seizures since childhood, each case is considered individually
Navy	Medical regulations state any attacks at any age would debar from entry
Air Force	Proven epilepsy (with a few exceptions) is a bar to recruitment. People developing epilepsy during service are given a medical employment standard that limits their employment
Coastguard	Coastguards come into a category that requires special physical qualifications; therefore medical examination is arranged in all cases to determine fitness to undertake the full range of duties
Diver	Any history of seizures (apart from febrile convulsions) will preclude granting a Certificate of Medical Fitness to Dive, which must be renewed every 12 months
Fire brigade	A history of epilepsy renders a person unsuitable for operational fire duties

Table 27
Continued

Occupation	Regulations
Merchant seamen	Absolute barrier on applicants with history of seizures since age 5. Serving seamen who develop epilepsy may be employed after 2 years free of seizures on a ship carrying a Medical Officer and provided they are not involved in the safety of ship or passengers
Nurse/midwife	Epilepsy is not mentioned specifically. Nurses: each training authority sets its own standards. Midwives: prospective trainees must provide evidence that they are not knowingly suffering from any disabilities that might preclude them from carrying out the duties of a midwife
Police	Applicants currently having seizures are not recruited. Those with past history dealt with on an individual basis. Also applies to traffic wardens, police drivers, etc.
Prison service	Recent history of epilepsy debars an applicant on grounds of security for posts at prison officer grade. Applicants to other grades of prison service are considered individually
Public transport driver/taxi driver	Absolute barrier if seizure occurred after attaining age of 5. Immediate loss of licence for existing licence holder
Teacher	Applicants must be 3 years free of seizures. Teachers in post may be barred from teaching physical education, craft, science and home economics
Train driver	Absolute barriers if seizure ever occurred or if seizure occurred since age 5

(From Craig and Oxley.)[99]

These regulations do not differentiate between auras, myoclonic jerks and more major seizures (all are counted as seizures) and they apply whether or not the patient is taking AEDs. Patients with a single seizure or other unexplained loss of consciousness may be barred from driving for a 12-month period, but someone with cerebral pathology (eg, a stroke or recent head injury) suffering a single seizure may be barred from driving for a 2-year period.

Clinicians should inform patients of these regulations and advise them of their responsibility to inform the DVLC, who will make the appropriate decision. Patients should be advised not to drive in the intervening period. Only in exceptional circumstances should a clinician consider contacting the DVLC about an individual patient.

Leisure activities

Any restrictions in leisure and sporting activities should be kept to a realistic minimum and will clearly vary according to a number of factors including:

(i)   the age of the person;
(ii) the specific epilepsy syndrome;
(iii) the degree of seizure control; and
(iv) the patient's interests and level of activities.

All too frequently there is the tendency to recommend that leisure and sports activities should be restricted and kept to a minimum, often with the statement, 'just in case something should happen'. There is no evidence for the often falsely held belief that epileptic seizures are more likely to occur during leisure or sporting activities, and in fact the converse may be true—that the threshold for seizures may be higher during sports and physical exercise.

Children. Restrictions and precautions will vary according to the child's seizure control and whether there are additional problems (eg, cerebral palsy or learning difficulties). However, for most children with uncomplicated and well-controlled epilepsy, there should be very few restrictions. Swimming should be encouraged, with the pool attendants or life guards simply being informed that the child has epilepsy.[101] Cycling (wearing a helmet) should also be encouraged, although preferably not on busy roads. In children with excellent seizure control there should arguably be no restrictions at all on games and activities (including most contact sports), although rock climbing may need to be considered carefully. Schools not uncommonly seek to impose restrictions on children with epilepsy, often through ignorance, but with good communication and advice schools will withdraw or relax any inappropriate restrictions.

Adults. Adults with epilepsy are subject to several statutory regulations that limit their activities; therefore it is important that additional unnecessary restrictions are not imposed by doctors, the public or, indeed, the patients themselves.

A decision as to whether to undertake any particular leisure activity should represent a balance between the risk of injury to the person with epilepsy or others and personal choice. Accordingly, the fewest restrictions apply to those whose epilepsy is in remission or in whom seizures occur only at predictable times (eg, in sleep or soon after waking).

In people with active epilepsy, certain high-risk activities should be avoided. These include parachuting, scuba diving and rock climbing.

People with epilepsy should never swim alone but swimming in public baths, with pool attendants aware of their condition, preferably but not necessarily accompanied, is to be encouraged. Like everyone else, people with epilepsy are advised to wear a helmet when cycling. With the exception of boxing there seems to be no particularly good reason to avoid contact sports.

A policy of disclosure of diagnosis is strongly recommended. Participation in any particular activity may have insurance implications for leisure activity organizers, who must never be 'kept in the dark'.

Allowing for the advice and suggestions above, most people with epilepsy can participate in most activities enjoyed by their non-epileptic peers.

Epilepsy clinics: Clinical nurse specialists in epilepsy

The management of epilepsy extends far beyond the prescription of antiepileptic medication. It is of course important to identify the type of epilepsy syndrome correctly and any underlying cause and to prescribe the most appropriate antiepileptic drug to obtain optimal control of seizures without side-effects. However, for many patients and their families, social, educational and psychological factors far outweigh the problem of preventing or controlling the seizures. This requires a multidisciplinary or 'team' approach, preferably within a specialist clinic, with education, support and advice from many different sources. Separate clinics should exist for children and adults. Members of the team should include:

- dedicated medical staff (interested and experienced in epilepsy)
- nurse specialist/liaison nurse in epilepsy
- clinical neuropsychologist
- psychiatrist (with a specific interest in learning difficulties)
- social worker
- representatives of the relevant local or national voluntary associations

The purpose of the clinic is to provide not only the best medical assessment and treatment, but also to provide a service that offers information, education, counselling and psychological support. There should be a specific psychological and psychiatric provision for patients with epilepsy, including those patients who have epilepsy in association with learning difficulties. The clinic should also provide a service for teenagers or adolescents with epilepsy, for whom follow-up in a children's hospital or unit is no longer appropriate; this would address the issues and concerns that are unique to this age group and allow a smooth hand-over of care from paediatric to adult services.

The epilepsy clinic cannot and should not exist in isolation; one of the key purposes of the clinic is to form a close link or liaison between the hospital and community health services (including school and family practice), and in so doing perhaps to reduce the unfortunate 'sick' or 'illness' stigma that is so often associated (or is perceived to be associated) with epilepsy.

The role of the clinical nurse specialist in epilepsy[102,103]

The clinical or liaison nurse specialist in epilepsy could be regarded as the pivotal team member in establishing the crucial hospital–community link and providing a management and education framework both for the primary health-care teams and for other professionals who may be involved (eg, teachers, educationalists, career information officers and employers).

The first epilepsy nurse liaison post in the UK was created in Doncaster in 1987. It focused on primary health-care teams. Since then the nurse specialist role has continued to evolve, with the establishment of the first nurse specialist based within a neuroscience unit in 1989 and the first paediatric nurse specialist post in 1992 (both in Liverpool). The Epilepsy Specialist Nurse Association (ESNA) was founded in 1991 by seven nurse specialists; this consequently raised the profile and role of the nurse specialists in the holistic management of epilepsy. In 1995, to mark the 45th anniversary of the British Epilepsy Association, the Association created a new nurse specialist post—the Sapphire Epilepsy Nurse. The current membership of ESNA is approximately 200.

The epilepsy nurse specialist has a role in the management of all people with epilepsy, but particularly of the following groups:

- parents of children with epilepsy
- teenagers with epilepsy
- women with epilepsy
- people with epilepsy and learning difficulties
- elderly people with epilepsy
- people with epilepsy who are contemplating surgical treatment

To meet the needs of these groups and the general population of all people with epilepsy, the nurse will offer information, support and counselling in many areas:

- the nature and causes of epilepsy
- the possible side-effects and interactions of any anti-epileptic drugs that have been prescribed
- contraception, pre-conception and pregnancy advice
- driving and DVLC regulations
- career choice and issues regarding employment and the disclosure of epilepsy
- sporting and leisure interests
- the effects of alcohol and recreational drugs on epilepsy and anti-epileptic drugs
- voluntary organizations

In undertaking this multi-faceted role the nurse must be able both to anticipate and to react to the changing circumstances of the patient with epilepsy (eg, addressing school-related issues, leaving school, relationships with peers and employers and family-planning).

Appendix:
Useful addresses

- **British Epilepsy Association**
  New Anstey House
  Gateway Drive
  Yeadon
  Leeds LS19 7XY
  Tel: (0113) 210 8800

- **National Information Centre**
  Tel: (0345) 089599

- **National Society for Epilepsy**
  Chalfont Centre
  Chalfont St Peter
  Buckinghamshire
  SL9 0RJ
  Tel: (01494) 873991

- **Epilepsy Association of Scotland**
  48 Govan Road
  Glasgow G5 1JL
  Tel: (0141) 427 4911

- **Irish Epilepsy Association**
  249 Crumlin Road
  Crumlin
  Dublin 12
  Tel: +353 1 557500

- **Mersey Region Epilepsy Association**
  The Glaxo Neurological Centre
  Norton Street
  Liverpool L3 8LR
  Tel: (0151) 298 2666

- **'Enlighten'**
  Action for Epilepsy
  5 Coates Place
  Edinburgh EH3 7AA
  Tel: (0131) 226 5458

References

1. Jackson JH (1873) On the anatomical, physiological and pathological investigation of epilepsies. *West Riding Lunatic Asylum Medical Reports 3:3:5*. Reprinted in Taylor J (ed.). *Selected Writings of John Hughlings Jackson*. Sevenoaks, Kent: Hodder and Stoughton. 1983, pp. 90–111.

2. Bernado LA and Pedley TA (1985) Cellular mechanisms of focal epileptogenesis. In *Recent Advances in Epilepsy, Vol. 2* (ed. Pedley TA and Meldrum BS). Edinburgh: Churchill Livingstone, pp. 21–36.

3. Gloor P (1988) Neurophysiological mechanism of generalised spike and wave discharge and its implications for understanding absence seizures. In *Elements of Petit Mal Epilepsy* (ed. Myslobodsky MS and Mirsky AF). New York: Peter Lang, pp. 159–210.

4. Ayala GF, Matsumoto H and Gumnit RJ (1970) Excitability changes and inhibitory mechanisms in neocortical neurones during seizures. *J Neurophysiol* **33**: 75–85.

5. Commission on Classification and Terminology of the International League Against Epilepsy (1981) Proposal for revised clinical and electroencephalographic classification of epileptic seizures. *Epilepsia* **22**: 489–501.

6. Commission on Classification and Terminology of the International League Against Epilepsy (1989) Proposal for classification of epilepsies and epileptic syndromes. *Epilepsia* **30**: 389–399.

7. Baxter P, Griffiths P, Kelly T and Gardner-Medwin D (1996) Pyridoxine dependent seizures: demographic, clinical, MRI and psychometric features and effect of dose on intelligence quotient. *Dev Med Child Neurol* **38**: 998–1006.

8. Tibbles JAR (1980) Dominant benign neonatal seizures. *Dev Med Child Neurol* **22**: 664–667.

9. Robinson R and Gardiner M (2000) Genetics of childhood epilepsy. *Arch Dis Child* **82**: 121–125.

10. Dravet C, Bureau M and Roger J (1992) Benign myoclonic epilepsy in infants. In *Epileptic Syndromes in Infancy, Childhood and Adolescence,* 2nd Ed (ed. Roger J, Dravet C, Bureau M, Dreifuss FE and Wolf P). London and Paris: John Libbey, pp. 67–74.

11. Appleton RE (1993) Infantile spasms. *Arch Dis Child* **69**: 614–618.

12. Livingston JH (1988) The Lennox–Gastaut syndrome. *Dev Med Child Neurol* **30**: 536–540.

13. Wolf SM (1979) Controversies in the treatment of febrile convulsions. *Neurology* **29**: 287–290.

14. Singh R, Scheffer IE, Crossland K and Berkovic SF (1999) Generalised epilepsy with febrile seizures plus: a common childhood-onset genetic epilepsy syndrome. *Ann Neurol* **45**: 75–81.

15. Loiseau P (1992) Childhood absence epilepsy. In *Epileptic Syndromes in Infancy, Childhood and Adolescence,* 2nd Ed (ed. Roger J, Dravet C, Bureau M, Dreifuss FE and Wolf P). London and Paris: John Libbey, pp. 135–150.

16. Berkovic SF, Andermann F, Carpenter S and Wolfe LS (1986) Progressive myoclonus epilepsies: specific causes and diagnosis. *N Engl J Med* **315**: 296–305.

17. Beaumanoir A (1992) The Landau–Kleffner syndrome. In *Epileptic Syndromes in Infancy, Childhood and Adolescence*, 2nd Ed (ed. Roger J, Dravet C, Bureau M, Dreifuss FE and Wolf P). London and Paris: John Libbey, pp. 231–243.

18. Wolf P (1992) Epilepsies with grand mal on wakening. In *Epileptic Syndromes in Infancy, Childhood and Adolescence*, 2nd Ed (ed. Roger J, Dravet C, Bureau M, Dreifuss FE and Wolf P). London and Paris: John Libbey, pp. 329–341.

19. Beaussart M (1972) Benign epilepsy of children with rolandic (centrotemporal) paroxysmal foci: a clinical entity: study of 221 cases. *Epilepsia* **13**: 795–811.

20. Janz D and Durner M (1997) Juvenile myoclonic epilepsy. In *Epilepsy: a Comprehensive Textbook* (ed. Engel J and Pedley TA). Philadelphia: Lippincott–Raven, pp. 2389–2400.

21. Oldani A, Zucconi M, Ferini-Strambini L *et al* (1996) Autosomal dominant nocturnal frontal lobe epilepsy: electroclinical picture. *Epilepsia* **37**: 964–976.

22. Appleton RE, Panayiotopoulos CP, Acomb BA and Beirne M (1993) Eyelid myoclonia with typical absences: an epilepsy syndrome. *J Neurol Neurosurg Psychiatry* **56**: 1312–1316.

23. Sander JWAS, Hart YM, Johnson AL and Shorvon S (1990) National General Practitioner Study of Epilepsy. Newly diagnosed epileptic seizures in the general population. *Lancet* **336**: 1267–1271.

24. Chadwick D, Cartlidge N and Bates D (1989). *Medical Neurology.* Edinburgh: Churchill Livingstone.

25. Binnie CD (1997) Simple reflex epilepsies. In *Epilepsy: a Comprehensive Textbook* (ed. Engel J and Pedley TA). Philadelphia: Lippincott-Raven, pp. 2489–2505.

26. Quirk JA, Fish DR, Smith SJM *et al* (1995) First seizures associated with playing electronic screen games: a community-based study in Great Britain. *Ann Neurol* **37**: 733–737.

27. Anderson VE, Hauser WA and Rich SS (1986) Genetic heterogeneity in the epilepsies. In *Advances in Neurology, Vol. 44* (ed. Delgado-Escueta AV, Ward Jr AA, Woodbury DM and Porter RJ). New York: Raven Press, pp. 59–75.

28. Hauser WA and Kurland LT (1975) The epidemiology of epilepsy in Rochester, Minnesota, 1935 through 1967. *Epilepsia* **16**: 1–66.

29. Hauser WA, Annegers JT and Elveback LR (1980) Mortality in patients with epilepsy. *Epilepsia* **21**: 399–412.

30. Nashef L, Brown SW (1997) Epilepsy and sudden death. *Epilepsia* **38 (suppl 11)**: S1–S76.

31. Commission for the Control of Epilepsy and its Consequences (1978) *Plan for Nationwide Action on Epilepsy, Vols 1–4*. DHEW Publications No. (NIH) 78–279. Bethesda, MD: US Department of Health Education and Welfare.

32. Shorvon SD (1988) Medical services. In *A Textbook of Epilepsy* (ed. Laidlaw J, Richens A and Oxley J). Edinburgh: Churchill Livingstone, pp. 611–630.

33. Meadow R (1984) Fictitious epilepsy. *Lancet* **ii**: 25–28.

34. Binnie CD and Prior PF (1994) Electroencephalography. *J Neurol Neurosurg Psychiatry* **57**: 308–319.

35. Smith D, Bartolo R, Pickles RM and Tedman BM. An audit of EEG requests in a district general hospital. Submitted to *BMJ*.

36. Kuzniecky RI and Jackson GD (1994) *MR in Epilepsy*. New York: Raven.

37. King MA, Newton MR, Jackson GD et al (1998) Epileptology of the first-seizure presentation: a clinical, EEG and MR imaging study of 300 consecutive patients. *Lancet* **352**: 1007–1011.

38. Smith D, Dafala B and Chadwick DW (1999) The misdiagnosis of epilepsy and the management of refractory epilepsy in a specialist clinic. *Q J Med* **92**: 15–23.

39. Lempert T, Bauer M and Schmidt D (1994) Syncope: a videometric analysis of 56 episodes of transient cerebral hypoxia. *Ann Neurol* **36**: 233–237.

40. Gibbs J and Appleton RE (1992) False diagnosis of epilepsy in children. *Seizure* **1**: 15–18.

41. Ellison PH, Largent JA and Behr JP (1981) A scoring system to predict outcome following neonatal seizures. *J Pediatr* **99**: 455–458.

42. Lombroso CT (1996) Neonatal seizures: a clinician's overview. *Brain Dev* **18**: 1–28.

43. Volpe JJ (1987) *Neurology of the Newborn*, 2nd Ed. Philadelphia: WB Saunders, pp. 144–146.

44. Nelson KB and Ellenberg JH (1976) Predictors of epilepsy in children who have febrile seizures. *N Engl J Med* **295**: 1029–1033.

45. Nelson KB and Ellenberg JH (1978) Prognosis in children with febrile seizures. *Pediatrics* **61**: 720–727.

46. Sell SHW (1983) Long-term sequelae of bacterial meningitis in children. *Pediatr Infect Dis* **2**: 90–93.

47. Ellenberg JH and Nelson KB (1984) Age of onset of seizures in young children. *Ann Neurol* **15**: 127–134.

48. Rosman NP, Peterson DB, Kaye EM and Colton T (1985) Seizures in bacterial meningitis: prevalence, patterns, pathogenesis and prognosis. *Pediatr Neurol* **1**: 278–285.

49. Annegers JF, Hauser WA, Beghi E, Nicolosi A and Kurland LT (1988) The risk of unprovoked seizures after encephalitis and meningitis. *Neurology* **38**: 1407–1410.

50. Bellman MH, Ross EM and Miller DL (1983) Infantile spasms and pertussis immunisation. *Lancet* **i**: 1031–1034.

51. Golden GS (1990) Pertussis vaccine and injury to the brain. *J Pediatr* **116**: 854–861.

52. Jennett B (1975) *Epilepsy after Non-Missile Head Injuries*, 2nd Ed. London: William Heinemann.

53. Annegers JF, Grabow JD, Groover RV, Laws ER, Elverback LA and Kurland LT (1980) Seizures after head trauma: a population study. *Neurology* (Minneap) **30**: 683–689.

54. Foy PM, Copeland GP and Shaw MDM (1981) The incidence of post operative seizures. *Acta Neurochir* **55**: 253–264.

55. Burn J (1990) *Epileptic Seizures after a First Stroke*. DM Thesis, Oxford University.

56. Berg AT and Shinnar S (1991) The risk of recurrence following a first unprovoked seizure. *Neurology* **41**: 965–972.

57. Chadwick D (1985) The discontinuation of antiepileptic therapy. In *Recent Advances in Epilepsy, Vol. 2* (ed. Meldrum BM and Pedley TA). Edinburgh: Churchill Livingstone.

58. MRC Antiepileptic Drug Withdrawal Study Group (1991) A randomised study of antiepileptic drug withdrawal in patients in remission of epilepsy. *Lancet* **337**: 1175–1180.

59. Jacoby A, Baker G, Chadwick D and Johnson A (1993) The impact of counselling with a practical statistical model on patients' decision-making about treatment for epilepsy. *Epilepsy Res* **16**: 207–214.

60. Chadwick D (1987) Overuse of monitoring of blood concentrations of antiepileptic drugs. *BMJ* **294**: 723–724.

61. Schmidt D (1982) *Adverse Effects of Antiepileptic Drugs*. New York: Raven Press.

62. Chadwick D (1988) The modern treatment of epilepsy. *Br J Hosp Med* **36**: 104–111.

63. Richens A (1991) The efficacy and safety of new anti-epileptic drugs. In *New Anti-epileptic Drugs* (ed. Pisani F, Perucca E, Avanzini G, Richens A). Amsterdam: Elsevier, pp. 89–98.

64. Brodie M, Richens A, Yuen AWC (1995) Double-blind comparison of lamotrigine and carbamazepine in newly diagnosed epilepsy. *Lancet* **345**: 476–479.

65. Marson AG, Kadir ZA, Hutton JL and Chadwick DW (1997) The new antiepileptic drugs: a systematic review of their efficacy and tolerability. *Epilepsia* **38**: 859–880.

66. Sachdeo RC, Reife RA, Lim P and Pledger G (1997) Topiramate monotherapy for partial onset seizures. *Epilepsia* **38**: 294–300.

67. Study of Standard And New Antiepileptic Drugs in the treatment of epilepsy (in press; details from the 'SANAD' Office, the Walton Centre for Neurology and Neurosurgery, Liverpool L9 7LJ).

68. Eke T, Talbot JF and Lawden MC (1997) Severe, persistent visual field constriction associated with vigabatrin. *BMJ* **314**: 180–181.

69. Lindhout D and Omitzigt JGC (1992) Pregnancy and the risk of teratogenicity. *Epilepsia* **35 (suppl 4)**: 541–548.

70. Clayton-Smith J and Donnai D (1995) Fetal valproate syndrome. *J Med Genet* **32:** 724–727.

71. Crawford P, Appleton R, Betts T, Duncan J, Guthrie E and Morrow J (The Women with Epilepsy Guidelines Development Group) (1999) Best practice guidelines for the management of women with epliepsy. *Seizure* **8**: 201–217.

72. Volpe JJ (1987) *Neurology of the Newborn.* 2nd Ed. Philadelphia: W.B. Saunders.

73. Rennie JM (1997) Neonatal seizures. *Eur J Pediatr* **156**: 83–87.

74. Freeman JM (1987) A clinical approach to the child with seizures and epilepsy. *Epilepsia* **28**: 103–109.

75. Stores G (1987) Pitfalls in the management of epilepsy. *Arch Dis Child* **62**: 88–90.

76. Matricardi M, Brinciotti M and Benedetti P (1989) Outcome after discontinuation of antiepileptic drug therapy in children with epilepsy. *Epilepsia* **30**: 582–589.

77. Kasteleijn-Nolst Trenité DA (1996) Cognitive aspects. In *Epilepsy in Children* (ed. Wallace S). London: Chapman and Hall Medical, pp. 581–599.

78. Vining E (1989) Educational, social and lifelong effects of epilepsy. *Pediatr Clin North Am* **36**: 449–461.

79. Richardson SA, Koller H, Katz M and McLaren J (1980) Seizures and epilepsy in a mentally retarded population over the first 22 years of life. *Appl Res Ment Retard* **1**: 123–138.

80. Corbett JA (1983) Epilepsy and mental retardation—a follow-up study. In *Advances in Epileptology: XIVth Epilepsy International Symposium* (ed. Parsonage M, Grant RHE, Craig AG and Ward AA). New York: Raven Press, pp. 203–214.

81. Leppik IF (1988) Management of seizures during pregnancy. In: *Recent Advances in Epilepsy, Vol. 4* (ed. Pedley TA and Meldrum BS). Edinburgh: Churchill Livingstone, pp. 109–121.

82. Tallis R (1989) Epilepsy in the elderly. In *IVth International Symposium on Sodium Valproate and Epilepsy* (ed. Chadwick D). London: Royal Society of Medicine, pp. 125–129.

83. Aminoff MJ and Simon RP (1980) Status epilepticus: causes, clinical features and consequences in 98 patients. *Am J Med* **69**: 657–666.

84. Howell SJL, Owen L and Chadwick DW (1989) Pseudostatus epilepticus. *Q J Med* **71**: 507–519.

85. Maytal J, Shinnar S, Moshe SL and Alvarez LA (1989) Low morbidity and mortality of status epilepticus in children. *Pediatrics* **83**: 323–331.

86. Graves NM and Kriel RL (1987) Rectal administration of anti-epileptic drugs in children. *Pediatr Neurol* **3**: 321–326.

87. Engel J (1993) *Surgical Treatment of the Epilepsies*, 2nd Ed. New York: Raven Press.

88. Huttenlocher RP (1976) Ketonemia and seizures: metabolic and anticonvulsant effects of two ketogenic diets in childhood epilepsy. *Pediatr Res* **10**: 536–540.

89. Schwartz RH, Eaton J, Aynsley-Green A and Bower BD (1983) Ketogenic diets in the management of childhood epilepsy. In *Research Progress in Epilepsy* (ed. Rose FC). London: Pitman, pp. 326–332.

90. Wheless JW (1995) The ketogenic diet: fa(c)t or fiction. *J Child Neurol* **10**: 419–423.

91. Vagus Nerve Stimulation Group (1995) A randomized controlled trial of chronic vagus nerve stimulation for treatment of medicinally intractable seizures. *Neurology* **45**: 224–230.

92. Schachter SC and Saper CB (1998) Progress in epilepsy research: vagus nerve stimulation. *Epilepsia* **39**: 677–686.

93. Bedini R, de Feo MR, Orano A and Rucchi L (1985) Effects of gamma-globulin therapy in severely epileptic children. *Epilepsia* **26**: 98–102.

94. Van Engelen BGM, Renier WO, Weemaes CMR, Gabreels FJM and Meinardi H (1994) Immunoglobulin treatment in epilepsy, a review of the literature. *Epilepsy Res* **19**: 181–190.

95. Aird RB (1983) The importance of seizure-inducing factors in the control of refractory forms of epilepsy. *Epilepsia* **24**: 567–583.

96. Feldman RG, Ricks NL and Orren NM (1983) Behavioural methods of seizure control. In *Epilepsy, Diagnosis and Management* (ed. Brown TR and Feldman RG). Boston: Little, Brown, pp. 269–279.

97. Whitman S and Hermann B (1986) *Psychopathology in Epilepsy: Social Dimensions.* Oxford: Oxford University Press.
98. Trimble MR and Reynold EH (1988) *Epilepsy, Behaviour and Congitive Functioning.* New York: John Wiley and Sons.
99. Craig A and Oxley J (1989) Social aspects of epilepsy. In *A Textbook of Epilepsy* (ed. Laidlaw J, Richens A and Oxley J). Edinburgh: Churchill Livingstone, pp. 566–610.
100. Taylor J, Chadwick D and Johnson T (1996) Risk of accidents in drivers with epilepsy. *J Neurol Neurosurg Psychiatry* **60**: 621–627.
101. Kemp AM and Sibert JR (1993) Epilepsy in children and the risk of drowning. *Arch Dis Child* **68**: 684–685.
102. Appleton RE and Sweeney A (1995) The management of epilepsy in children: the role of the clinical nurse specialist. *Seizure* **4**: 287–291.
103. Risdale L (2000) The effect of specially trained epilepsy nurses in primary care: a review. *Seizure* **9**: 43–46.

Index